The World's Best Anatomical Charts:

Diseases & Disorders

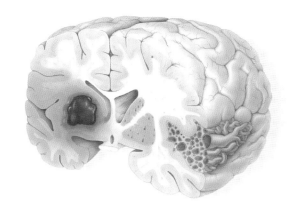

"The World's Best Anatomical Charts: Diseases and Disorders" groups together 36 of our best selling charts. Concentrating on many common disorders and diseases of the body, this book features our most popular titles as well as current additions to our collection of world famous charts.

Our team of certified medical illustrators, consultants and physicians develop each chart to ensure accuracy, clarity and timeliness of subject. All of the charts have been digitally enhanced to bring you the best reproduction quality, and have been updated and revised with terminology and illustrations that reflect the most current medical advances.

Each chart is clearly labeled and easy to read. The desk-sized format makes this collection handy for the study of human anatomy, patient consultation or quick reference.

Diseases and Disorders illustrations include cardiovascular disease, cancer, hypertension, asthma, and epilepsy. Everyday conditions and ailments such as allergies and the common cold are included, as well as topics in the forefront of medicine today such as Parkinson's Disease, Alzheimer's, and G.E.R.D. Each chart is presented in a clear and concise manner, explaining causes, symptoms and physiologies. Using "The World's Best Anatomical Charts: Diseases and Disorders" in combination with our book, "The World's Best Anatomical Charts: Systems and Structures," gives you access to the most complete and easy-to-use medical reference of charts in today's market.

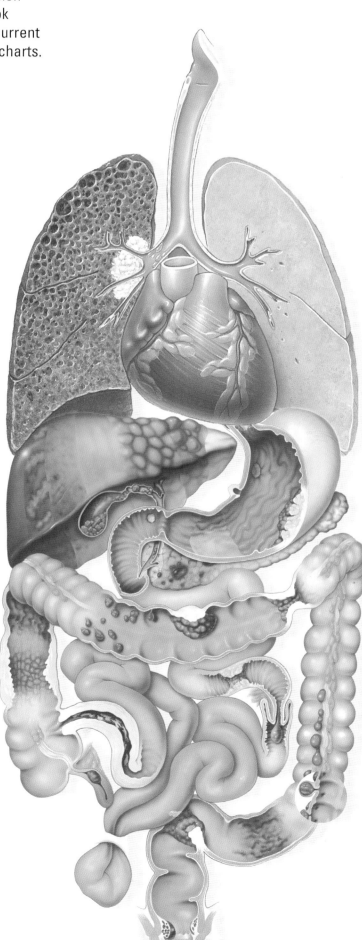

Table of Contents

GASTROESOPHAGEAL DISORDERS AND DIGESTIVE ANATOMY

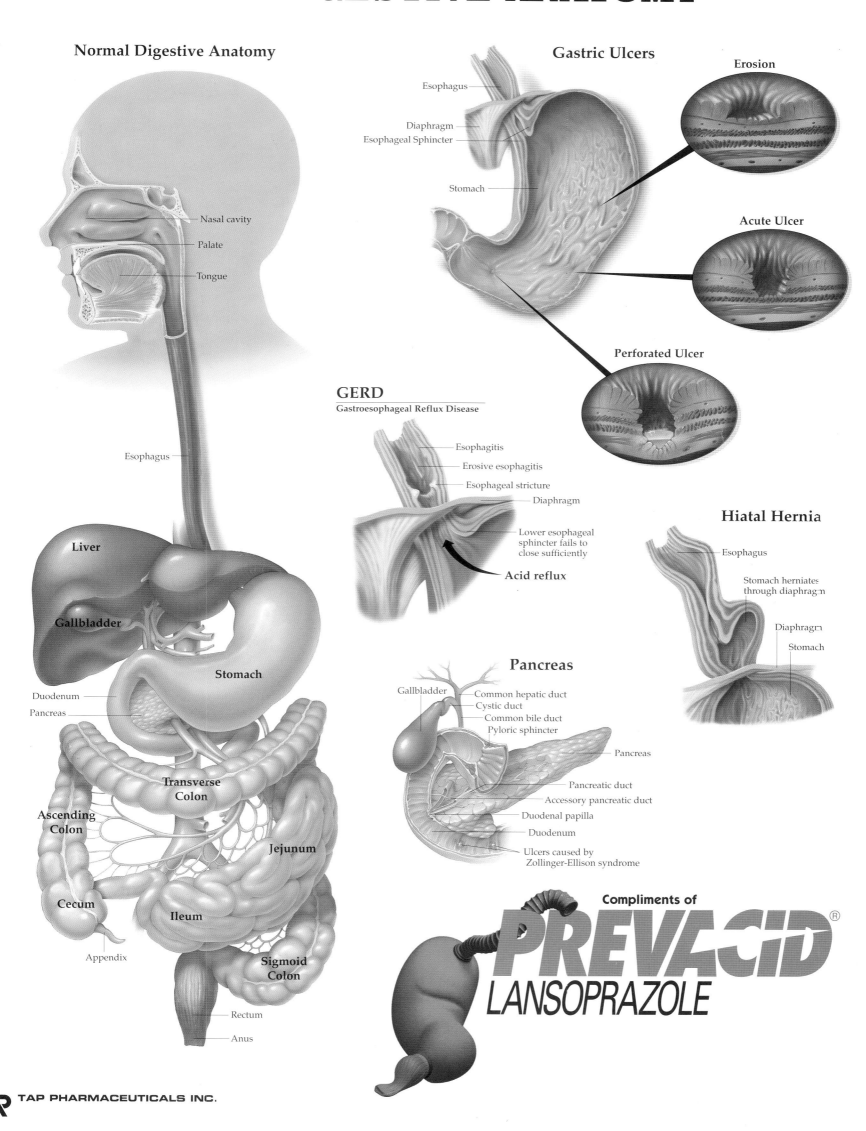

Normal Digestive Anatomy

Nasal cavity
Palate
Tongue
Esophagus
Liver
Gallbladder
Stomach
Duodenum
Pancreas
Transverse Colon
Ascending Colon
Jejunum
Cecum
Ileum
Appendix
Sigmoid Colon
Rectum
Anus

Gastric Ulcers

Esophagus
Diaphragm
Esophageal Sphincter
Stomach

Erosion

Acute Ulcer

Perforated Ulcer

GERD
Gastroesophageal Reflux Disease

Esophagitis
Erosive esophagitis
Esophageal stricture
Diaphragm
Lower esophageal sphincter fails to close sufficiently
Acid reflux

Hiatal Hernia

Esophagus
Stomach herniates through diaphragm
Diaphragm
Stomach

Pancreas

Gallbladder
Common hepatic duct
Cystic duct
Common bile duct
Pyloric sphincter
Pancreas
Pancreatic duct
Accessory pancreatic duct
Duodenal papilla
Duodenum
Ulcers caused by Zollinger-Ellison syndrome

Compliments of

PREVACID®
LANSOPRAZOLE

TAP PHARMACEUTICALS INC.

For further information, including adverse events, please see the accompanying complete prescribing information for PREVACID.

1

DESORDENES GASTROESOFAGICOS Y ANATOMÍA DIGESTIVA

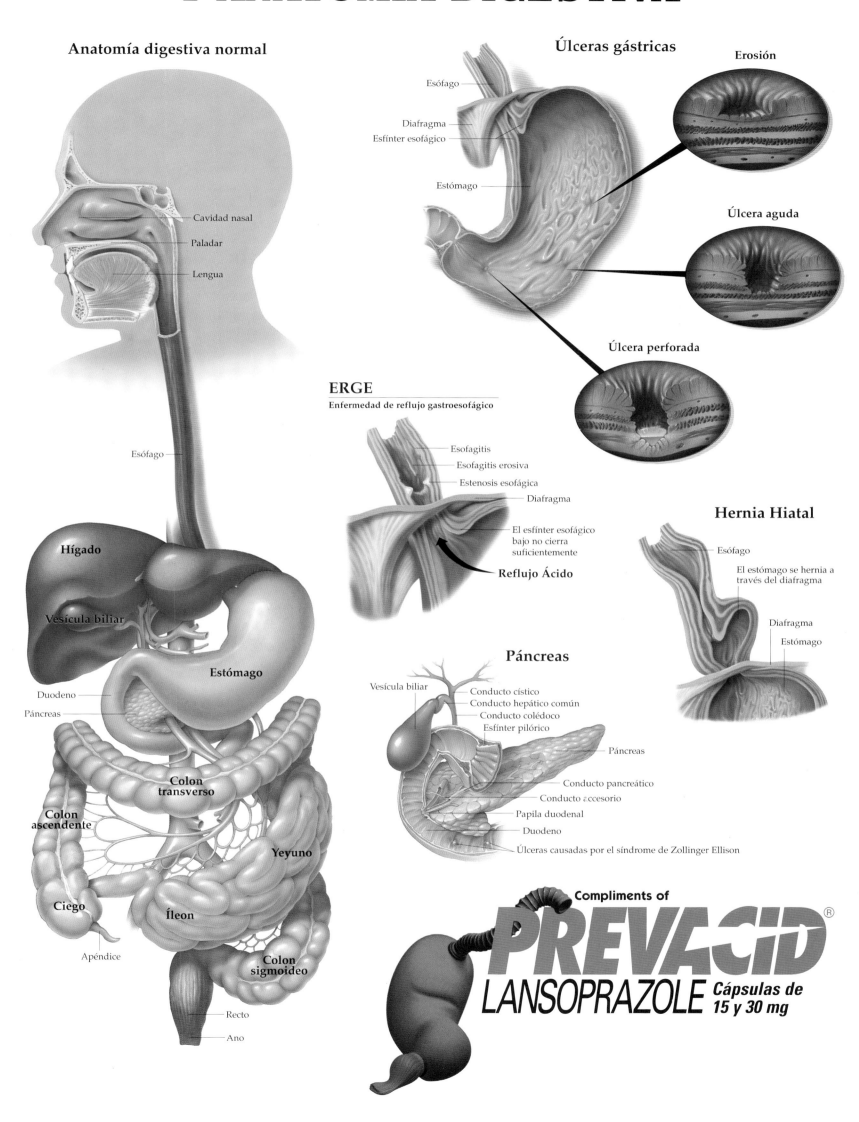

Anatomía digestiva normal

- Cavidad nasal
- Paladar
- Lengua
- Esófago
- Hígado
- Vesícula biliar
- Estómago
- Duodeno
- Páncreas
- Colon transverso
- Colon ascendente
- Yeyuno
- Ciego
- Íleon
- Apéndice
- Colon sigmoideo
- Recto
- Ano

Úlceras gástricas

- Esófago
- Diafragma
- Esfínter esofágico
- Estómago

Erosión

Úlcera aguda

Úlcera perforada

ERGE
Enfermedad de reflujo gastroesofágico

- Esofagitis
- Esofagitis erosiva
- Estenosis esofágica
- Diafragma
- El esfínter esofágico bajo no cierra suficientemente

Reflujo Ácido

Hernia Hiatal

- Esófago
- El estómago se hernia a través del diafragma
- Diafragma
- Estómago

Páncreas

- Vesícula biliar
- Conducto cístico
- Conducto hepático común
- Conducto colédoco
- Esfínter pilórico
- Páncreas
- Conducto pancreático
- Conducto accesorio
- Papila duodenal
- Duodeno
- Úlceras causadas por el síndrome de Zollinger Ellison

Compliments of

PREVACID®
LANSOPRAZOLE Cápsulas de 15 y 30 mg

DANGERS OF ALCOHOL

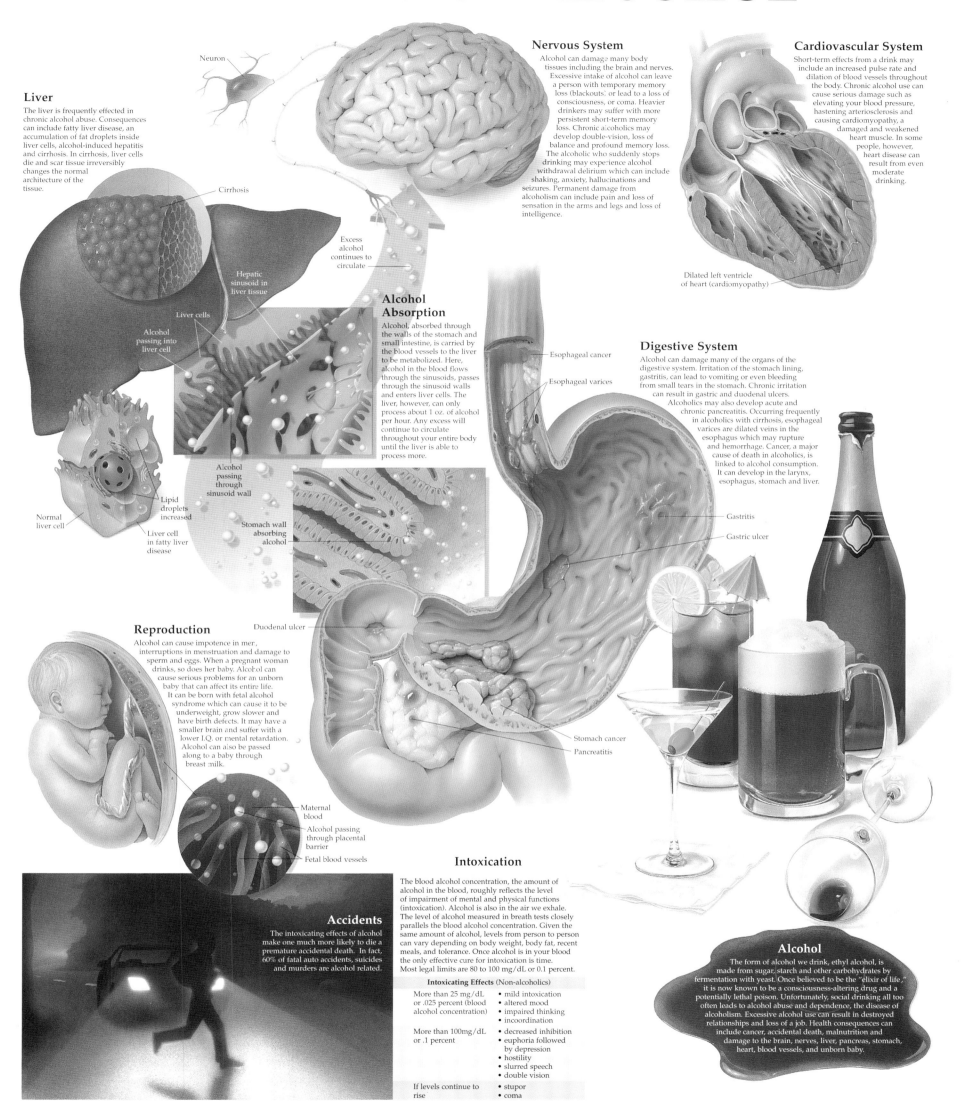

Liver

The liver is frequently effected in chronic alcohol abuse. Consequences can include fatty liver disease, an accumulation of fat droplets inside liver cells, alcohol-induced hepatitis and cirrhosis. In cirrhosis, liver cells die and scar tissue irreversibly changes the normal architecture of the tissue.

Cirrhosis

Hepatic sinusoid in liver tissue

Liver cells

Alcohol passing into liver cell

Normal liver cell

Lipid droplets increased

Liver cell in fatty liver disease

Alcohol passing through sinusoid wall

Stomach wall absorbing alcohol

Nervous System

Alcohol can damage many body tissues including the brain and nerves. Excessive intake of alcohol can leave a person with temporary memory loss (blackouts) or lead to a loss of consciousness, or coma. Heavier drinkers may suffer with more persistent short-term memory loss. Chronic alcoholics may develop double-vision, loss of balance and profound memory loss. The alcoholic who suddenly stops drinking may experience alcohol withdrawal delirium which can include shaking, anxiety, hallucinations and seizures. Permanent damage from alcoholism can include pain and loss of sensation in the arms and legs and loss of intelligence.

Neuron

Excess alcohol continues to circulate

Cardiovascular System

Short-term effects from a drink may include an increased pulse rate and dilation of blood vessels throughout the body. Chronic alcohol use can cause serious damage such as elevating your blood pressure, hastening arteriosclerosis and causing cardiomyopathy, a damaged and weakened heart muscle. In some people, however, heart disease can result from even moderate drinking.

Dilated left ventricle of heart (cardiomyopathy)

Alcohol Absorption

Alcohol, absorbed through the walls of the stomach and small intestine, is carried by the blood vessels to the liver to be metabolized. Here, alcohol in the blood flows through the sinusoids, passes through the sinusoid walls and enters liver cells. The liver, however, can only process about 1 oz. of alcohol per hour. Any excess will continue to circulate throughout your entire body until the liver is able to process more.

Digestive System

Alcohol can damage many of the organs of the digestive system. Irritation of the stomach lining, gastritis, can lead to vomiting or even bleeding from small tears in the stomach. Chronic irritation can result in gastric and duodenal ulcers. Alcoholics may also develop acute and chronic pancreatitis. Occurring frequently in alcoholics with cirrhosis, esophageal varices are dilated veins in the esophagus which may rupture and hemorrhage. Cancer, a major cause of death in alcoholics, is linked to alcohol consumption. It can develop in the larynx, esophagus, stomach and liver.

Esophageal cancer

Esophageal varices

Gastritis

Gastric ulcer

Stomach cancer

Pancreatitis

Duodenal ulcer

Reproduction

Alcohol can cause impotence in men, interruptions in menstruation and damage to sperm and eggs. When a pregnant woman drinks, so does her baby. Alcohol can cause serious problems for an unborn baby that can affect its entire life. It can be born with fetal alcohol syndrome which can cause it to be underweight, grow slower and have birth defects. It may have a smaller brain and suffer with a lower I.Q. or mental retardation. Alcohol can also be passed along to a baby through breast milk.

Maternal blood

Alcohol passing through placental barrier

Fetal blood vessels

Accidents

The intoxicating effects of alcohol make one much more likely to die a premature accidental death. In fact, 60% of fatal auto accidents, suicides and murders are alcohol related.

Intoxication

The blood alcohol concentration, the amount of alcohol in the blood, roughly reflects the level of impairment of mental and physical functions (intoxication). Alcohol is also in the air we exhale. The level of alcohol measured in breath tests closely parallels the blood alcohol concentration. Given the same amount of alcohol, levels from person to person can vary depending on body weight, body fat, recent meals, and tolerance. Once alcohol is in your blood the only effective cure for intoxication is time. Most legal limits are 80 to 100 mg/dL or 0.1 percent.

Intoxicating Effects (Non-alcoholics)

More than 25 mg/dL or .025 percent (blood alcohol concentration)	• mild intoxication • altered mood • impaired thinking • incoordination
More than 100mg/dL or .1 percent	• decreased inhibition • euphoria followed by depression • hostility • slurred speech • double vision
If levels continue to rise	• stupor • coma

Alcohol

The form of alcohol we drink, ethyl alcohol, is made from sugar, starch and other carbohydrates by fermentation with yeast. Once believed to be the "elixir of life," it is now known to be a consciousness-altering drug and a potentially lethal poison. Unfortunately, social drinking all too often leads to alcohol abuse and dependence, the disease of alcoholism. Excessive alcohol use can result in destroyed relationships and loss of a job. Health consequences can include cancer, accidental death, malnutrition and damage to the brain, nerves, liver, pancreas, stomach, heart, blood vessels, and unborn baby.

©1998, 2000 Anatomical Chart Company, a division of Springhouse Corporation.
Medical illustrations by Kimberly A. Martens, in consultation with David Yu, M.D.

9696

3

UNDERSTANDING ALLERGIES

What Is an Allergy?

An allergy is an acquired sensitivity of the immune system. This means that the body's immune system has become sensitive to one or more common, ordinarily harmless substances in our environment, such as pollen, dust, molds or even food. This sensitivity causes an immune response which results in symptoms that range from mild (runny nose, watery eyes, sneezing, and itching) or severe (hives, trouble breathing, or anaphylactic shock). Symptoms usually occur with each exposure to the allergen.

Allergens

An allergen is a general term used to describe something that causes an allergic reaction. Allergens are actually tiny proteins found on certain substances. Some examples are airborne allergens, like pollen and mold or foods like shellfish, peanuts and milk. Venom from an insect sting contains allergens, as do plants like poison ivy. Allergens also exist indoors, like dust mites. Only those who are prone to acquired sensitivity are regularly affected by these allergens.

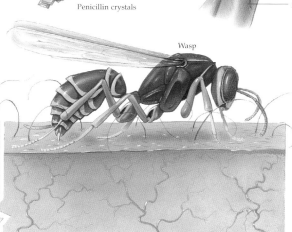

Pollen grains

Pet dander

Penicillin crystals

Hair

Anaphylaxis: An Allergic Emergency

Anaphylaxis is a life-threatening reaction. The onset of this reaction occurs within seconds or minutes of exposure. Symptoms include red raised blotches over most of the body. Skin becomes warm to the touch, intense tightening and swelling of the airways make breathing difficult, and there is a drop in blood pressure. Breathing can stop and the body may slip into shock. If medication is not administered quickly, heart failure and death can result within minutes. Allergens in insect venom and injectable medications are more likely to cause anaphylaxis than are any other allergens. Anaphylaxis is not a common reaction and can be controlled with prompt medication and the help of a physician.

Pathway of an Allergic Reaction

Two phases exists in allergic reactions, primary exposure and re-exposure. In this example, the primary exposure is from allergens in the venom of an insect sting.

Wasp

Wasp

The Immune System

The immune system relies on two types of white blood cells, called T-cells and B-cells. These cells help the immune system defend the body by recognizing foreign and potentially harmful substances, and then releasing potent chemicals to combat the foreign invaders. An allergic reaction occurs when the immune system mistakenly recognizes a harmless substance (such as pollen) and becomes sensitive to that substance. Repeated exposures to the substance, even years later, can trigger an allergic reaction.

Who Gets Allergies?

The tendency to develop allergies is thought to be inherited, because they commonly develop in those who have a family history of allergies. However, it is possible for anyone to develop allergies at any age. Environmental factors can make our immune systems overly sensitive. This could then trigger allergies in people with no family history or hasten the onset in those with a family history.

Primary Exposure

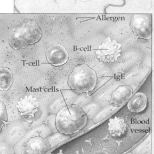

Allergen

B-cell

T-cell

IgE

Mast cells

Blood vessel

T-cells recognize the foreign allergen and release chemicals that instruct B-cells to produce millions of antibodies, called immunoglobulin E (IgE). (Each time a different type of allergen triggers IgE production, a new type of IgE is produced, specific to that allergen). IgE's then attach themselves to mast cells. Mast cells with attached IgE's can remain in the body for years, ready to react to the same allergen.

Re-exposure

With re-exposure, allergens re-enter the body and directly contact the IgE antibodies attached to the mast cells. This stimulates the mast cells to quickly release chemicals such as histamine. The release of these chemicals can cause tightening of smooth muscles in the airways; dilation of small blood vessels (resulting in warming and swelling of skin tissues); increased mucus secretion in the nasal cavity and airways; and itching.

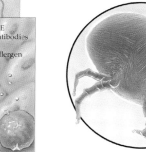

Mast cell

IgE antibodies

Allergen

Histamine and other chemicals

Household Allergies

Dust mites are microscopic organisms that live on skin tissue that is shed off regularly. The mites are commonly found on pillows, mattresses, upholstered furniture and in clothes-changing areas. These organisms are responsible for most of the year-round type of allergic rhinitis or "hay fever."

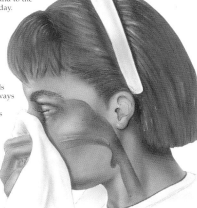

Dust mite

Insect Allergies

Venom injected by wasps and bees contain allergens that can cause an allergic reaction in 1 out of 10 people. Those not allergic to insect stings or bites experience normal swelling and skin irritation that last for a few hours. Those with insect allergies tend to have large areas of hives, swelling and itching that may last for days or weeks. However, for others, the reaction can develop into a life-threatening emergency called anaphylactic shock. Anyone with a sensitivity to stings or bites should see an allergist for diagnosis and treatment.

Wasps, bees, hornets and yellow jackets, which belong to the order Hymenoptera, are responsible for many cases of insect allergies each year.

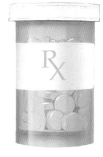

Yellow jacket

Hornet

Drug Allergies

Drug allergies are not common, but they can produce uncomfortable and life-threatening reactions. Penicillin allergy can cause symptoms ranging from mild rashes to anaphylactic shock within minutes. Other drugs that may cause allergic reactions are antibiotics, sulfa drugs, anti-epileptic drugs and insulin.

Respiratory Allergies

Allergies of the respiratory system are the most common types of allergies. This may be due to the large number of immune cells located along the respiratory tract and to the many potential allergens inhaled every day. The most common inhaled allergens are from pollen, molds, dust mites, and pet dander. Hay fever and asthma are types of respiratory allergies.

Hay fever, or allergic rhinitis, is a common allergy. It is usually associated with the pollen season. The immune cells lining the nose, sinuses, eyelids and airways are very sensitive to airborne allergens, such as pollen from ragweed. Symptoms of hay fever include runny nose, sneezing, watery eyes and itchy throat. These symptoms usually occur every year at about the same time and last at least as long as the pollen is produced.

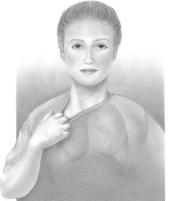

Asthma is a condition in which there is tightening, swelling and increased mucus secretion in the airways in the lungs. This causes difficulty breathing, plus wheezing and tightening of the chest. It is most common in children and can be a mild or life-threatening reaction. This condition can be caused by inhaling allergens such as pollen, pet dander and dust; however, not all asthma is related to allergies. It can also be triggered by irritants such as tobacco smoke.

Skin Allergies

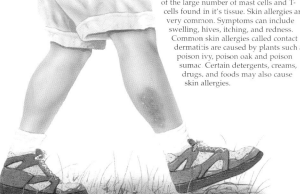

Skin protects us from the environment. Exposed daily to a variety of allergens, skin is especially sensitive to allergens because of the large number of mast cells and T-cells found in it's tissue. Skin allergies are very common. Symptoms can include swelling, hives, itching, and redness. Common skin allergies called contact dermatitis are caused by plants such as poison ivy, poison oak and poison sumac. Certain detergents, creams, drugs, and foods may also cause skin allergies.

Food Allergies

Allergies to foods can cause swelling of the lips, throat, face and tongue; upset stomach, vomiting, cramps; hives; eczema — even asthma. Some common food allergens are milk, soy, eggs, peanuts, wheat, fish and shellfish. Food allergies are most common in childhood but can also occur in adults.

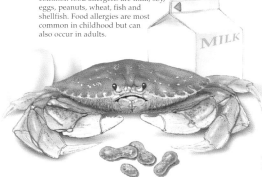

MILK

Managing Allergies

The first step to managing allergies is to identify what type of reaction you're having, whether it is watery eyes, sneezing or difficulty breathing.

Secondly, try to identify the trigger or the situation which led to the symptoms. Ask a few question:

Where did the reaction occur?
Inside or outside?
Were you eating or drinking?
Were there any animals or insects near you?
Were you wearing something new?
Or did you use a new soap or detergent?

A physician can perform an allergy test with a variety of common allergens. Once the allergen has been identified, manage your allergies by following some tips:

- Avoid allergens when possible,
- Avoid tobacco smoke and other irritants,
- Use medication as prescribed,
- See a doctor regularly,
- Stay healthy.

©1997, 1999, 2000 Anatomical Chart Company, a division of Springhouse Corporation.
Medical illustrations by Marcelo Oliver, in consultation with Jacqueline Pongracic, M.D.

9864

4

UNDERSTANDING ALZHEIMER'S

The Aging Brain and Dementia

At birth, the brain contains as many nerve cells, called **neurons**, as it will ever have — many billions of neurons! Unlike other cells of our body, such as skin or bone, neurons cannot reproduce themselves. Therefore, as we age, neurons that die from normal wear and tear and injury are not replaced. The normal effects of aging can cause mild forgetfulness and slowed reflexes. However, there are diseases, known as **dementias**, that in their early stages mimic these age-related changes. Dementia is characterized by the dramatic decline of intellectual function.

Dementia's most common form is Alzheimer's Disease (AD), a slowly progressive disorder that destroys the neurons and communication pathways of the brain. It is the fourth leading cause of death in adults in the U.S. and is perhaps the most devastating chronic disease for patients and their families. AD usually strikes those over the age of 65; the average course of the disease is 6 to 10 years from onset. Although the causes of AD are largely unknown, in some cases genetic factors are responsible.

At present there is no reliable diagnostic test for AD. The physician must eliminate any other reversible causes of dementia, such as problems caused by medications or other diseases. A comprehensive medical history is taken, and a general and neurologic examination as well as laboratory tests are performed. Only after other potential causes have been identified, treated, or eliminated can a diagnosis of probable AD be made.

Abnormal Cellular Structures

How and why neurons die in AD is largely unknown. However, several characteristic abnormal cellular structures, which scientists believe cause cell malfunction or cell death, are found in the brain of every AD patient. These structures include excessive granulovacuoles, neurofibrillary tangles, and amyloid plaques.

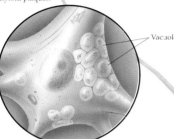

Vacuoles

Granulovacuolar degeneration

is found inside the neurons of the hippocampus. An abnormally high number of fluid-filled spaces, called **vacuoles**, enlarge the cell's body, possibly causing the cell to malfunction or die.

Normal Neuron

Dendrites

Neurofilament

Nucleus

Vacuole

Cell body

Axon

message

Neurotransmitters: The Messengers

AD also destroys the way some neurons "talk" to each other. Neurons communicate via a chemical message that passes between two cells across a tiny gap called a **synapse**. A neuron receives messages from its **dendrites** and passes the information to the **cell body**, where the message is received. The message can then be sent to the end of the axon, where sacs containing chemicals called **neurotransmitters** are released. The sacs empty the neurotransmitter into the synapse between the two cells. The chemical message is picked up by the other cell and the process continues.

Groups of neurons that use the same neurotransmitter form specialized network systems. Several of these systems are damaged in AD. One in particular, the cholinergic system, uses the neurotransmitter acetylcholine to send its messages. The relay center for this system, the nucleus basalis of Meynert, suffers severe neuron loss and decreased production of acetylcholine. This is believed to play a role in loss of memory.

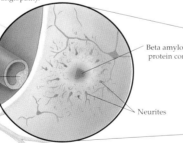

message

Neurotransmitter (acetylcholine)

Dendrite of receiving neuron

Receptor site

Synapse

Sacs containing neurotransmitter

Axon

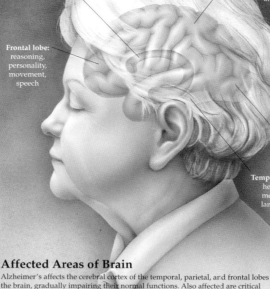

Hippocampus: memory and learning

Parietal lobe: language, sense of temperature, touch, pain, and space

Frontal lobe: reasoning, personality, movement, speech

Occipital lobe: vision

Temporal lobe: hearing, memory, language

Affected Areas of Brain

Alzheimer's affects the cerebral cortex of the temporal, parietal, and frontal lobes of the brain, gradually impairing their normal functions. Also affected are critical structures deep inside the brain that process and relay information to the cerebral cortex and other areas. Those structures include the **hippocampus**, which processes short-term memory, the **amygdala**, which controls emotional drives (anger, sex, fear), and the **nucleus basalis of Meynert**, which is a relay center of neurons using the neurotransmitter acetylcholine (see Neurotransmitters: The Messengers).

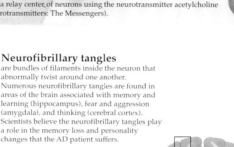

Neurofibrillary tangles

are bundles of filaments inside the neuron that abnormally twist around one another. Numerous neurofibrillary tangles are found in areas of the brain associated with memory and learning (hippocampus), fear and aggression (amygdala), and thinking (cerebral cortex). Scientists believe the neurofibrillary tangles play a role in the memory loss and personality changes that the AD patient suffers.

Tangles

Amyloid plaques

(senile plaques) are found outside neurons in the extracellular space of the cerebral cortex and hippocampus. Amyloid plaques contain a core of **beta amyloid protein** that is surrounded by abnormal nerve endings, or **neurites**. Amyloid also occurs in the walls of cerebral blood vessels, causing the condition called amyloid angiopathy.

Beta amyloid protein core

Amyloid in blood vessel

Neurites

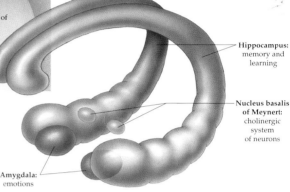

Hippocampus: memory and learning

Nucleus basalis of Meynert: cholinergic system of neurons

Amygdala: emotions

Cerebral cortex (grey matter): thinking

Stages of Alzheimer's Disease

Managing AD involves two important considerations: first, enabling patients to be as independent as possible, maintaining their quality of life, and second, providing support for the family. By understanding the general stages of AD, patients and their families can plan for the future.

Stage I: Early or Mild Phase
Early signs are continual forgetfulness and difficulty recalling new names and recent conversations. Personality changes may appear, such as decreased motivation and drive, or becoming easily upset or anxious. Patients may become disoriented or lost in familiar surroundings. Some early symptoms go unnoticed because the patient's social skills cover up these difficulties.

Stage II: Middle or Moderate Phase
Memory worsens, especially with current events. Some patients may become depressed, withdrawn, or agitated. Patients may require help in decision making and managing personal finances. Overall, the patient depends more on others for daily care.

Stage III: Late or Severe Phase
The patient is usually unaware of time and place, and, at times, cannot identify close family members. Patients may become increasingly insecure, suspicious, and agitated. Sleep may be disturbed, and movement and coordination may become slower and more difficult. The patient requires constant care for daily functions, requiring many families to seek nursing home care for their loved one.

Physical Changes in the Cortex

White matter

Neuron cell body

Axon

Alzheimer's   Normal

The brain is formed of two tissue types known as grey and white matter. The grey matter, in the **cerebral cortex**, is the outer brain tissue that contains neuron cell bodies. The axons of the neurons extend deep into the inner tissue, or white matter, to form pathways connecting the different functional areas of the brain. When large numbers of neurons are damaged, gaps occur in communication, severely limiting one's ability to think and remember. In AD the greatest loss of neurons occurs in the cortex of the temporal and parietal lobes, causing the grey matter of that area to shrink, or atrophy.

Management of Alzheimer's Disease

Although there is no cure for AD, medical and community resources are available to patients and their families. Local chapters of the Alzheimer's Association offer counseling and support-group programs for families. In addition, local respite and adult-care programs offer help. The physician may also prescribe drugs to treat the emotional and cognitive symptoms of AD. Consult your physician for more information, or contact your local Alzheimer's Association chapter or the national Alzheimer's Association referral service at 1-800-272-3900.

©1995, 2000 Anatomical Chart Company, a division of Springhouse Corporation.
Written and illustrated by Tonya Hines, CMI, inconsultation with Peter J. Whitehouse, M.D., Ph.D.

9976

ARTHRITIS-JOINT INFLAMMATION

There are over 100 different forms of arthritis. The following are the most common:

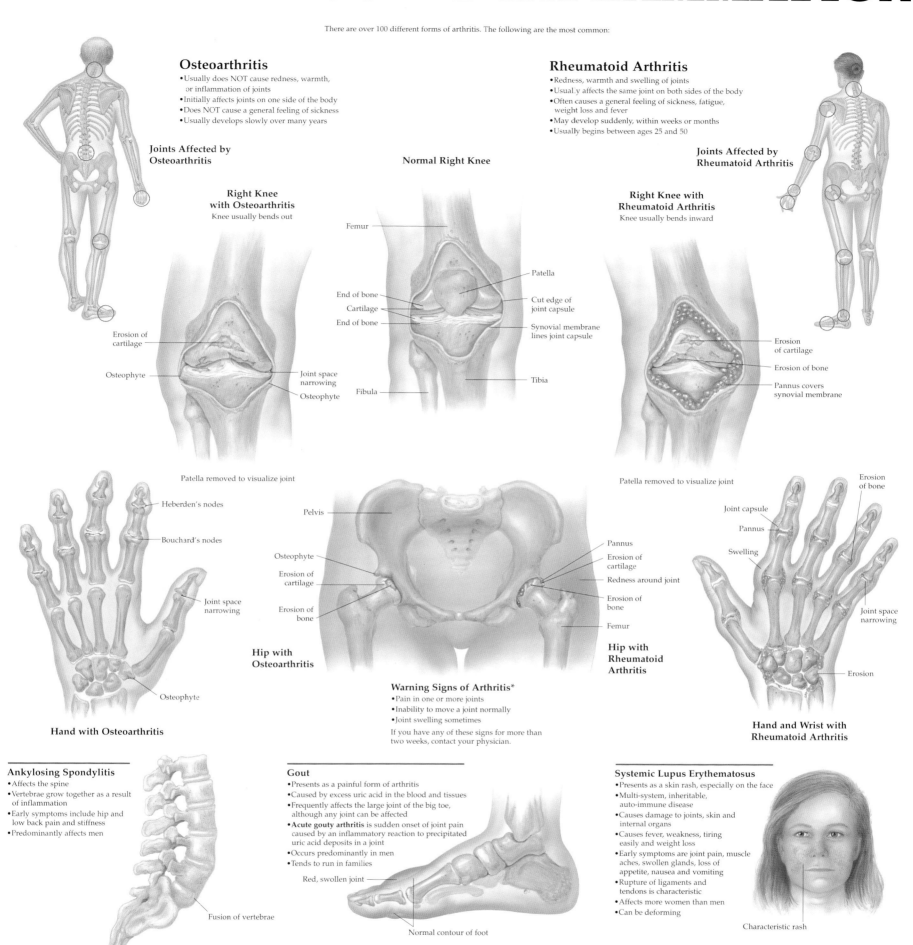

Osteoarthritis
- Usually does NOT cause redness, warmth, or inflammation of joints
- Initially affects joints on one side of the body
- Does NOT cause a general feeling of sickness
- Usually develops slowly over many years

Rheumatoid Arthritis
- Redness, warmth and swelling of joints
- Usually affects the same joint on both sides of the body
- Often causes a general feeling of sickness, fatigue, weight loss and fever
- May develop suddenly, within weeks or months
- Usually begins between ages 25 and 50

Joints Affected by Osteoarthritis

Normal Right Knee

Joints Affected by Rheumatoid Arthritis

Right Knee with Osteoarthritis
Knee usually bends out

Erosion of cartilage
Osteophyte
Joint space narrowing
Osteophyte

Right Knee with Rheumatoid Arthritis
Knee usually bends inward

Femur
Patella
End of bone
Cartilage
End of bone
Cut edge of joint capsule
Synovial membrane lines joint capsule
Fibula
Tibia

Erosion of cartilage
Erosion of bone
Pannus covers synovial membrane

Patella removed to visualize joint

Patella removed to visualize joint

Hand with Osteoarthritis

Heberden's nodes
Bouchard's nodes
Joint space narrowing
Osteophyte

Hip with Osteoarthritis

Pelvis
Osteophyte
Erosion of cartilage
Erosion of bone

Hip with Rheumatoid Arthritis

Pannus
Erosion of cartilage
Redness around joint
Erosion of bone
Femur

Hand and Wrist with Rheumatoid Arthritis

Erosion of bone
Joint capsule
Pannus
Swelling
Joint space narrowing
Erosion

Warning Signs of Arthritis*
- Pain in one or more joints
- Inability to move a joint normally
- Joint swelling sometimes

If you have any of these signs for more than two weeks, contact your physician.

Ankylosing Spondylitis
- Affects the spine
- Vertebrae grow together as a result of inflammation
- Early symptoms include hip and low back pain and stiffness
- Predominantly affects men

Fusion of vertebrae

Gout
- Presents as a painful form of arthritis
- Caused by excess uric acid in the blood and tissues
- Frequently affects the large joint of the big toe, although any joint can be affected
- **Acute gouty arthritis** is sudden onset of joint pain caused by an inflammatory reaction to precipitated uric acid deposits in a joint
- Occurs predominantly in men
- Tends to run in families

Red, swollen joint
Normal contour of foot

Systemic Lupus Erythematosus
- Presents as a skin rash, especially on the face
- Multi-system, inheritable, auto-immune disease
- Causes damage to joints, skin and internal organs
- Causes fever, weakness, tiring easily and weight loss
- Early symptoms are joint pain, muscle aches, swollen glands, loss of appetite, nausea and vomiting
- Rupture of ligaments and tendons is characteristic
- Affects more women than men
- Can be deforming

Characteristic rash

Related Disorders

Fibromyalgia (Fibrositis)
- A form of rheumatoid disease
- Presents as fatigue and pain in muscles, ligaments and tendons
- NOT a form of arthritis
- Does not cause deformity
- People who develop fibromyalgia frequently have unfit or poorly developed muscles
- Sleep disturbances are common

Myofascial Pain
- Results from the strain or improper use of a muscle
- Starts and stops suddenly
- Pain is worse at rest than during exercise

Bursitis
- Inflammation of a bursa, a small fluid-filled sac that absorbs shock and reduces friction around a joint
- May be caused by physical stress on a joint
- Starts suddenly and ends within a few days to weeks

Tendinitis
- Inflammation of a tendon, a cord of fibrous tissue that attaches muscle to bone
- May be caused by physical stress on a tendon
- Starts suddenly and ends within a few days or weeks

Shoulder

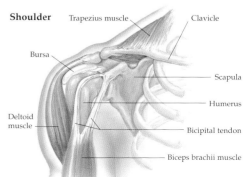

Trapezius muscle
Clavicle
Bursa
Scapula
Humerus
Deltoid muscle
Bicipital tendon
Biceps brachii muscle

©1992, 1997, 1999, 2000 Anatomical Chart Company, a division of Springhouse Corporation.
Medical illustrations by Linda Warren, in consultation with Judith L. Thrall, R.N., and John L. Skosey, M.D., Ph.D., Professor of medicine and Chief, section of Rheumatology, The University of Illinois Hospitals and Clinics.

UNDERSTANDING BREAST DISEASE

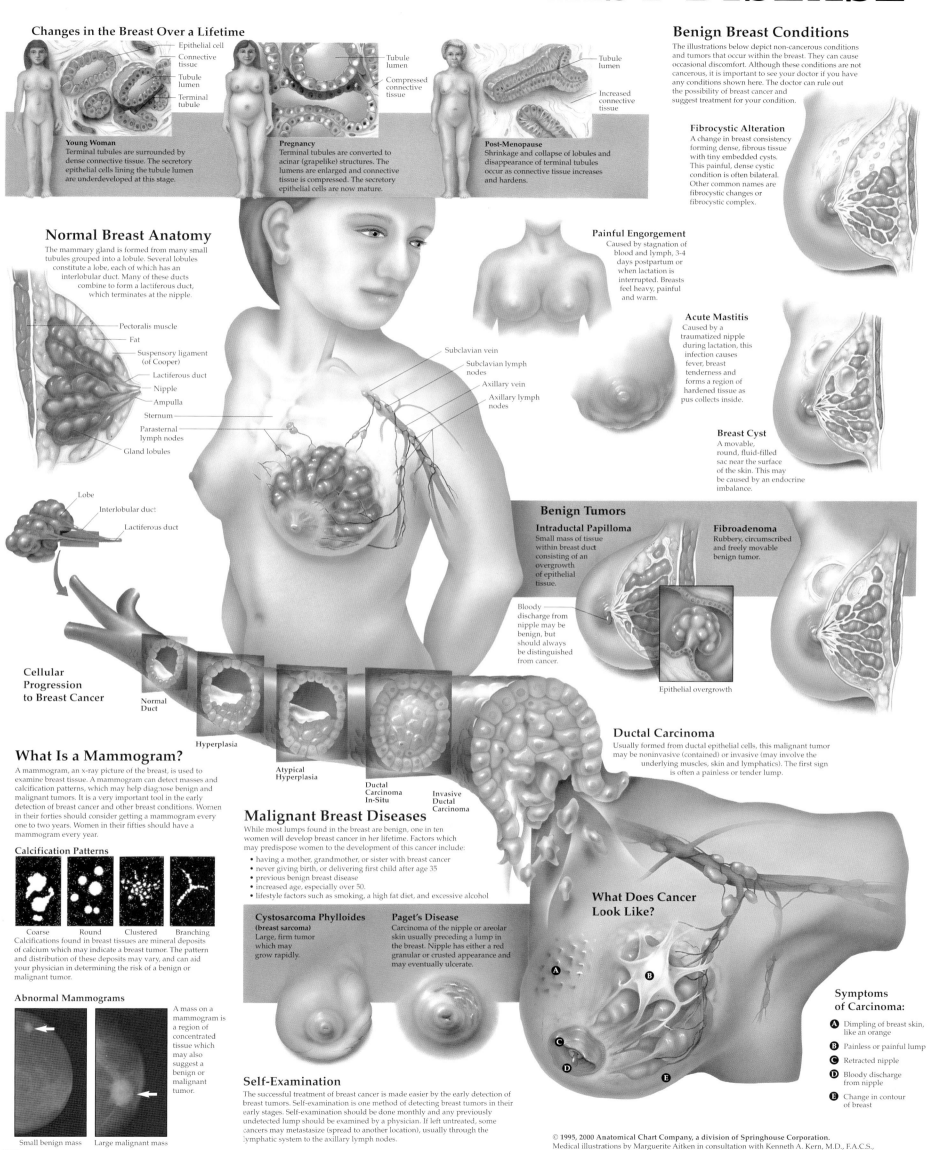

Changes in the Breast Over a Lifetime

Epithelial cell
Connective tissue
Tubule lumen
Terminal tubule

Young Woman
Terminal tubules are surrounded by dense connective tissue. The secretory epithelial cells lining the tubule lumen are underdeveloped at this stage.

Tubule lumen
Compressed connective tissue

Pregnancy
Terminal tubules are converted to acinar (grapelike) structures. The lumens are enlarged and connective tissue is compressed. The secretory epithelial cells are now mature.

Tubule lumen
Increased connective tissue

Post-Menopause
Shrinkage and collapse of lobules and disappearance of terminal tubules occur as connective tissue increases and hardens.

Benign Breast Conditions

The illustrations below depict non-cancerous conditions and tumors that occur within the breast. They can cause occasional discomfort. Although these conditions are not cancerous, it is important to see your doctor if you have any conditions shown here. The doctor can rule out the possibility of breast cancer and suggest treatment for your condition.

Fibrocystic Alteration
A change in breast consistency forming dense, fibrous tissue with tiny embedded cysts. This painful, dense cystic condition is often bilateral. Other common names are fibrocystic changes or fibrocystic complex.

Normal Breast Anatomy

The mammary gland is formed from many small tubules grouped into a lobule. Several lobules constitute a lobe, each of which has an interlobular duct. Many of these ducts combine to form a lactiferous duct, which terminates at the nipple.

Pectoralis muscle
Fat
Suspensory ligament (of Cooper)
Lactiferous duct
Nipple
Ampulla
Sternum
Parasternal lymph nodes
Gland lobules

Subclavian vein
Subclavian lymph nodes
Axillary vein
Axillary lymph nodes

Painful Engorgement
Caused by stagnation of blood and lymph, 3-4 days postpartum or when lactation is interrupted. Breasts feel heavy, painful and warm.

Acute Mastitis
Caused by a traumatized nipple during lactation, this infection causes fever, breast tenderness and forms a region of hardened tissue as pus collects inside.

Breast Cyst
A movable, round, fluid-filled sac near the surface of the skin. This may be caused by an endocrine imbalance.

Lobe
Interlobular duct
Lactiferous duct

Benign Tumors

Intraductal Papilloma
Small mass of tissue within breast duct consisting of an overgrowth of epithelial tissue.

Bloody discharge from nipple may be benign, but should always be distinguished from cancer.

Epithelial overgrowth

Fibroadenoma
Rubbery, circumscribed and freely movable benign tumor.

Cellular Progression to Breast Cancer

Normal Duct
Hyperplasia
Atypical Hyperplasia
Ductal Carcinoma In-Situ
Invasive Ductal Carcinoma

Ductal Carcinoma
Usually formed from ductal epithelial cells, this malignant tumor may be noninvasive (contained) or invasive (may involve the underlying muscles, skin and lymphatics). The first sign is often a painless or tender lump.

What Is a Mammogram?

A mammogram, an x-ray picture of the breast, is used to examine breast tissue. A mammogram can detect masses and calcification patterns, which may help diagnose benign and malignant tumors. It is a very important tool in the early detection of breast cancer and other breast conditions. Women in their forties should consider getting a mammogram every one to two years. Women in their fifties should have a mammogram every year.

Calcification Patterns

Coarse
Round
Clustered
Branching

Calcifications found in breast tissues are mineral deposits of calcium which may indicate a breast tumor. The pattern and distribution of these deposits may vary, and can aid your physician in determining the risk of a benign or malignant tumor.

Abnormal Mammograms

A mass on a mammogram is a region of concentrated tissue which may also suggest a benign or malignant tumor.

Small benign mass
Large malignant mass

9757

Malignant Breast Diseases

While most lumps found in the breast are benign, one in ten women will develop breast cancer in her lifetime. Factors which may predispose women to the development of this cancer include:

• having a mother, grandmother, or sister with breast cancer
• never giving birth, or delivering first child after age 35
• previous benign breast disease
• increased age, especially over 50.
• lifestyle factors such as smoking, a high fat diet, and excessive alcohol

Cystosarcoma Phylloides
(breast sarcoma)
Large, firm tumor which may grow rapidly.

Paget's Disease
Carcinoma of the nipple or areolar skin usually preceding a lump in the breast. Nipple has either a red granular or crusted appearance and may eventually ulcerate.

What Does Cancer Look Like?

Ⓐ
Ⓑ
Ⓒ
Ⓓ
Ⓔ

Symptoms of Carcinoma:

Ⓐ Dimpling of breast skin, like an orange

Ⓑ Painless or painful lump

Ⓒ Retracted nipple

Ⓓ Bloody discharge from nipple

Ⓔ Change in contour of breast

Self-Examination

The successful treatment of breast cancer is made easier by the early detection of breast tumors. Self-examination is one method of detecting breast tumors in their early stages. Self-examination should be done monthly and any previously undetected lump should be examined by a physician. If left untreated, some cancers may metastasize (spread to another location), usually through the lymphatic system to the axillary lymph nodes.

UNDERSTANDING CANCER

What is Cancer?

Cancer is a destructive (malignant) growth of cells which invades nearby tissues and may metastasize (spread) to other areas of the body. Dividing rapidly, these cells tend to be very aggressive and out of control. In contrast, a benign tumor is simply a localized mass of slowly multiplying cells resembling its original tissue and are seldom life-threatening.

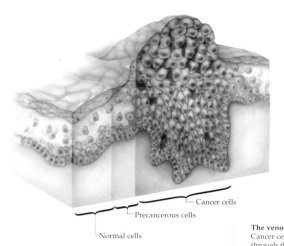

Cancer cells
Precancerous cells
Normal cells

What is a Carcinogen?

Factors found in the environment which may increase the risk of cancer are called carcinogens. These include:

- Cigarette Smoking
- Exposure to industrial agents and chemicals
- Radiation
- Pollution
- Alcohol
- Some viruses
- Sun exposure

Most experts believe that repeated or long term exposure to these elements damages normal cells. Heredity is another factor which plays a role in the risk of breast, colon and skin cancer.

The Diagnosis

Most benign cells are considered harmless unless their size or location threaten nearby structures. Any sign of cancer should be detected and treated early for a better chance of a full recovery. The diagnosis of malignant cancer is determined by a microscopic examination of sampled (biopsied) tissue. Measuring the extent the cells have spread, called **staging**, can be done using a variety of imaging techniques. Computerized Axial Tomography (CAT-scan) is a rotating X-ray machine used to take cross-sectional pictures of specific tumors. Magnetic Resonance Imaging (MRI) uses a magnetic field and radiofrequency waves to make detailed images of some parts of the body, like the brain.

The four stages of malignant cancer are determined by the spread of the cancer cells. This classification helps physicians develop a treatment plan specific to each individual cancer.

How Does Cancer Spread?

Cancer cells may invade nearby tissues or metastasize (spread) to other organs. There are three ways in which cancer cells may move to other tissues:

The venous system: Cancer cells may travel through the veins, often to the liver and the lungs.

Middle colic vein
Superior mesenteric artery and vein
Ascending colon
Transverse colon
Lymph nodes
Primary cancer

The lymphatic system: Cancer cells may move through this series of channels from the tissues to lymph nodes and eventually to the circulatory system.

Seeding: Cancer may penetrate an organ, moving into a body cavity (chest or abdominal space) and spread throughout that area.

Cancer Incidence by Site and Sex

(based on information from the American Cancer Society)
*Excluding nonmelanoma skin cancer and carcinoma in situ.

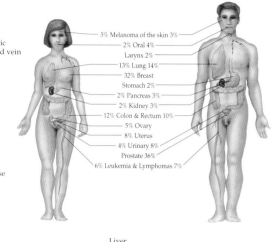

3% Melanoma of the skin 3%
2% Oral 4%
Larynx 2%
13% Lung 14%
32% Breast
Stomach 2%
2% Pancreas 3%
2% Kidney 3%
12% Colon & Rectum 10%
5% Ovary
8% Uterus
4% Urinary 8%
Prostate 36%
6% Leukemia & Lymphomas 7%

Liver
Lymph nodes
Pancreas
Metastatic cancer
Bile duct
Lymph nodes
Primary cancer

Stage IV:
Metastasis (spread) of the tumor occurs in other tissues of the body.

Cancer
Epithelium
Dermis

Stage I:
The cancer is small, localized and limited.

Lymph nodes
Metastatic cancer
Primary cancer
Mammary ducts
Mammary glands

Stage II:
Local spreading occurs in the organ and lymph nodes.

Metastatic cancer in lymph nodes
Aorta
Left lung

Stage III:
Cancer cells invade neighboring tissues and lymph nodes.

Cancer Treatments

Due to the variety of cancers, the ideal treatment can range from observation to complicated surgical removal with aggressive therapy. Surgery, radiation therapy and chemotherapy can be used in combination or as individual treatments. Some cancers may also be treated with hormone or biological therapy which can be described by a physician. Successful treatment may lead to remission (a condition when signs of the disease are gone).

Surgery

As a method of local treatment, the diseased part of the body is removed. Neighboring healthy lymph nodes and tissues may also be removed to help control the spread of the cancer.

Radiation Therapy

High energy rays, focused in a beam, are used to damage the cancer cells and stop their reproduction. This local therapy is used to shrink a cancer's size either before surgical removal or after, to kill any remaining cancer cells. Side effects may range from minimal to moderate including: tiredness, skin rashes, and a decrease in infection-fighting white blood cells.

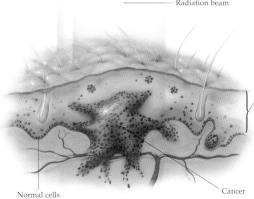

Radiation beam
Epithelium
Normal cells
Cancer

Chemotherapy

Synthetic drugs, given at prearranged, timed intervals, are used to disrupt a cancer cell's ability to grow. These drugs act, via the blood, on the entire body. In addition to treating the cancer, they may cause temporary side effects in fast growing cells like those of the blood, stomach and hair. Common side effects are hair loss, nausea, vomiting and a reduced number of white blood cells. These side effects increase the chance of infection.

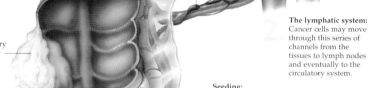

Capillary
Normal cells
Cancer cells
Chemotherapy
Red blood cell

Achieving a Healthy Lifestyle

Understanding cancer and its cause is the best way to develop a healthier lifestyle and avoid exposure to its risks. Some preventative measures include:

- Selecting a balanced diet high in fiber, low in fat.
- Limiting alcohol intake.
- Maintaining low body fat.
- Doing self examinations.
- Getting regular check-ups.

It is very important to follow your physician's instructions and to seek the support of family and friends. Cancer-related support groups are also available to discuss issues surrounding cancer.

9756

CARDIOVASCULAR DISEASE

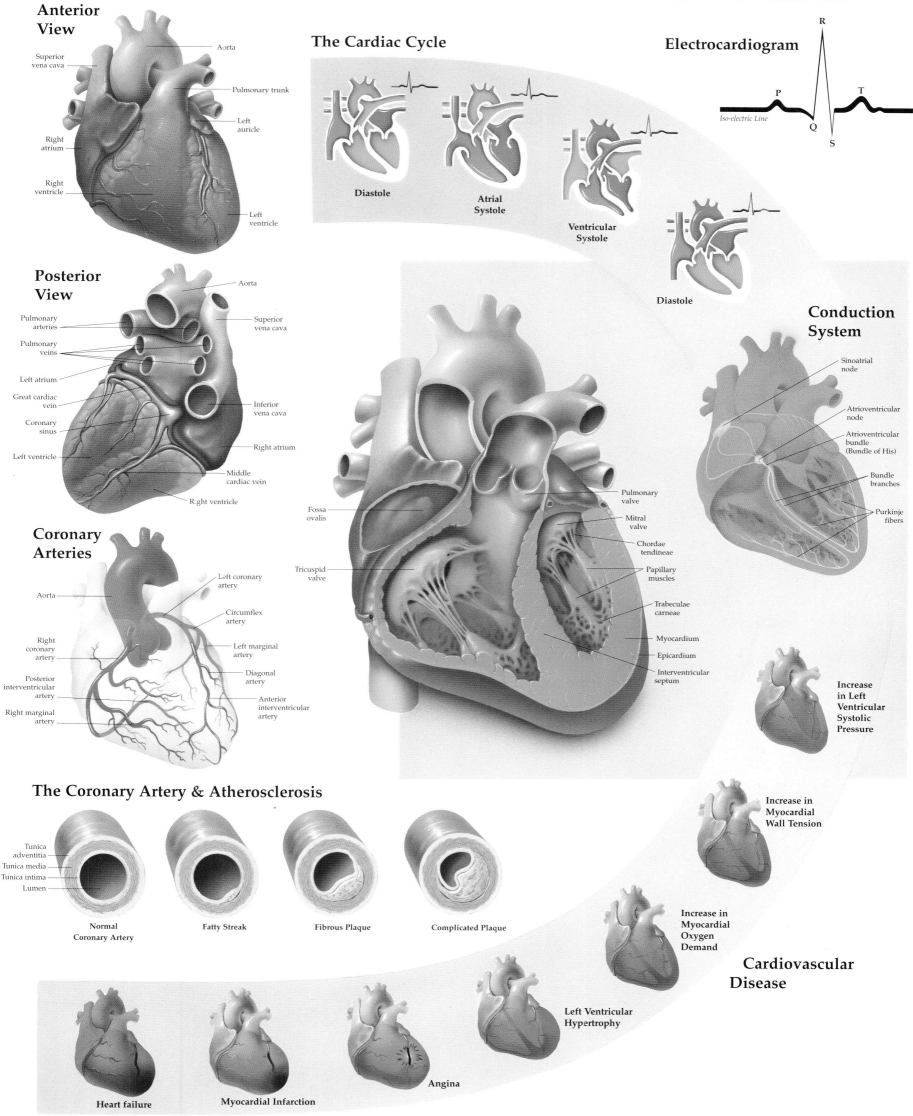

Anterior View

- Aorta
- Superior vena cava
- Pulmonary trunk
- Left auricle
- Right atrium
- Right ventricle
- Left ventricle

Posterior View

- Aorta
- Pulmonary arteries
- Superior vena cava
- Pulmonary veins
- Left atrium
- Great cardiac vein
- Coronary sinus
- Inferior vena cava
- Left ventricle
- Right atrium
- Middle cardiac vein
- Right ventricle

Coronary Arteries

- Left coronary artery
- Circumflex artery
- Aorta
- Left marginal artery
- Right coronary artery
- Diagonal artery
- Posterior interventricular artery
- Anterior interventricular artery
- Right marginal artery

The Cardiac Cycle

- Diastole
- Atrial Systole
- Ventricular Systole
- Diastole

Electrocardiogram

- R
- P
- T
- Q
- S
- Iso-electric Line

- Fossa ovalis
- Tricuspid valve
- Pulmonary valve
- Mitral valve
- Chordae tendineae
- Papillary muscles
- Trabeculae carneae
- Myocardium
- Epicardium
- Interventricular septum

Conduction System

- Sinoatrial node
- Atrioventricular node
- Atrioventricular bundle (Bundle of His)
- Bundle branches
- Purkinje fibers

- Increase in Left Ventricular Systolic Pressure
- Increase in Myocardial Wall Tension
- Increase in Myocardial Oxygen Demand
- Left Ventricular Hypertrophy

Cardiovascular Disease

The Coronary Artery & Atherosclerosis

- Tunica adventitia
- Tunica media
- Tunica intima
- Lumen

- Normal Coronary Artery
- Fatty Streak
- Fibrous Plaque
- Complicated Plaque

- Heart failure
- Myocardial Infarction
- Angina

9915

UNDERSTANDING CARPAL TUNNEL SYNDROME

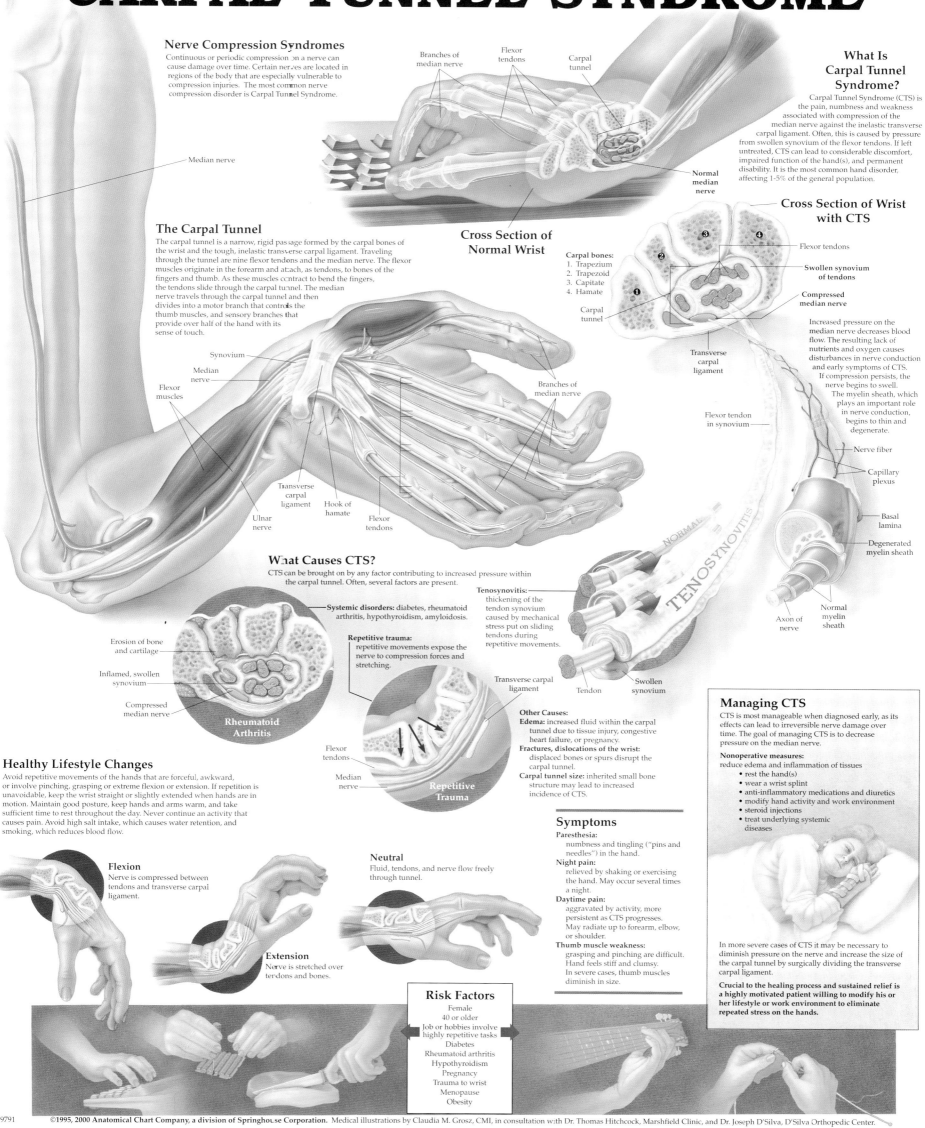

Nerve Compression Syndromes

Continuous or periodic compression on a nerve can cause damage over time. Certain nerves are located in regions of the body that are especially vulnerable to compression injuries. The most common nerve compression disorder is Carpal Tunnel Syndrome.

Median nerve

Branches of median nerve
Flexor tendons
Carpal tunnel

Normal median nerve

What Is Carpal Tunnel Syndrome?

Carpal Tunnel Syndrome (CTS) is the pain, numbness and weakness associated with compression of the median nerve against the inelastic transverse carpal ligament. Often, this is caused by pressure from swollen synovium of the flexor tendons. If left untreated, CTS can lead to considerable discomfort, impaired function of the hand(s), and permanent disability. It is the most common hand disorder, affecting 1-5% of the general population.

The Carpal Tunnel

The carpal tunnel is a narrow, rigid passage formed by the carpal bones of the wrist and the tough, inelastic transverse carpal ligament. Traveling through the tunnel are nine flexor tendons and the median nerve. The flexor muscles originate in the forearm and attach, as tendons, to bones of the fingers and thumb. As these muscles contract to bend the fingers, the tendons slide through the carpal tunnel. The median nerve travels through the carpal tunnel and then divides into a motor branch that controls the thumb muscles, and sensory branches that provide over half of the hand with its sense of touch.

Synovium
Median nerve
Flexor muscles
Transverse carpal ligament
Hook of hamate
Flexor tendons
Ulnar nerve
Branches of median nerve

Cross Section of Normal Wrist

Carpal bones:
1. Trapezium
2. Trapezoid
3. Capitate
4. Hamate

Carpal tunnel

Cross Section of Wrist with CTS

Flexor tendons
Swollen synovium of tendons
Compressed median nerve
Transverse carpal ligament

Increased pressure on the median nerve decreases blood flow. The resulting lack of nutrients and oxygen causes disturbances in nerve conduction and early symptoms of CTS. If compression persists, the nerve begins to swell. The myelin sheath, which plays an important role in nerve conduction, begins to thin and degenerate.

Flexor tendon in synovium
Nerve fiber
Capillary plexus
Basal lamina
Degenerated myelin sheath
Axon of nerve
Normal myelin sheath

What Causes CTS?

CTS can be brought on by any factor contributing to increased pressure within the carpal tunnel. Often, several factors are present.

Systemic disorders: diabetes, rheumatoid arthritis, hypothyroidism, amyloidosis.

Repetitive trauma: repetitive movements expose the nerve to compression forces and stretching.

Erosion of bone and cartilage
Inflamed, swollen synovium
Compressed median nerve

Rheumatoid Arthritis

Flexor tendons
Median nerve

Repetitive Trauma

Tenosynovitis: thickening of the tendon synovium caused by mechanical stress put on sliding tendons during repetitive movements.

Transverse carpal ligament
Tendon
Swollen synovium

TENOSYNOVITIS

Other Causes:
Edema: increased fluid within the carpal tunnel due to tissue injury, congestive heart failure, or pregnancy.
Fractures, dislocations of the wrist: displaced bones or spurs disrupt the carpal tunnel.
Carpal tunnel size: inherited small bone structure may lead to increased incidence of CTS.

Healthy Lifestyle Changes

Avoid repetitive movements of the hands that are forceful, awkward, or involve pinching, grasping or extreme flexion or extension. If repetition is unavoidable, keep the wrist straight or slightly extended when hands are in motion. Maintain good posture, keep hands and arms warm, and take sufficient time to rest throughout the day. Never continue an activity that causes pain. Avoid high salt intake, which causes water retention, and smoking, which reduces blood flow.

Flexion
Nerve is compressed between tendons and transverse carpal ligament.

Extension
Nerve is stretched over tendons and bones.

Neutral
Fluid, tendons, and nerve flow freely through tunnel.

Symptoms

Paresthesia:
numbness and tingling ("pins and needles") in the hand.
Night pain:
relieved by shaking or exercising the hand. May occur several times a night.
Daytime pain:
aggravated by activity, more persistent as CTS progresses. May radiate up to forearm, elbow, or shoulder.
Thumb muscle weakness:
grasping and pinching are difficult. Hand feels stiff and clumsy. In severe cases, thumb muscles diminish in size.

Managing CTS

CTS is most manageable when diagnosed early, as its effects can lead to irreversible nerve damage over time. The goal of managing CTS is to decrease pressure on the median nerve.

Nonoperative measures:
reduce edema and inflammation of tissues
- rest the hand(s)
- wear a wrist splint
- anti-inflammatory medications and diuretics
- modify hand activity and work environment
- steroid injections
- treat underlying systemic diseases

In more severe cases of CTS it may be necessary to diminish pressure on the nerve and increase the size of the carpal tunnel by surgically dividing the transverse carpal ligament.

Crucial to the healing process and sustained relief is a highly motivated patient willing to modify his or her lifestyle or work environment to eliminate repeated stress on the hands.

Risk Factors

Female
40 or older
Job or hobbies involve highly repetitive tasks
Diabetes
Rheumatoid arthritis
Hypothyroidism
Pregnancy
Trauma to wrist
Menopause
Obesity

9791   ©1995, 2000 Anatomical Chart Company, a division of Springhouse Corporation. Medical illustrations by Claudia M. Grosz, CMI, in consultation with Dr. Thomas Hitchcock, Marshfield Clinic, and Dr. Joseph D'Silva, D'Silva Orthopedic Center.

CONDITIONS FOR CESAREAN SECTION

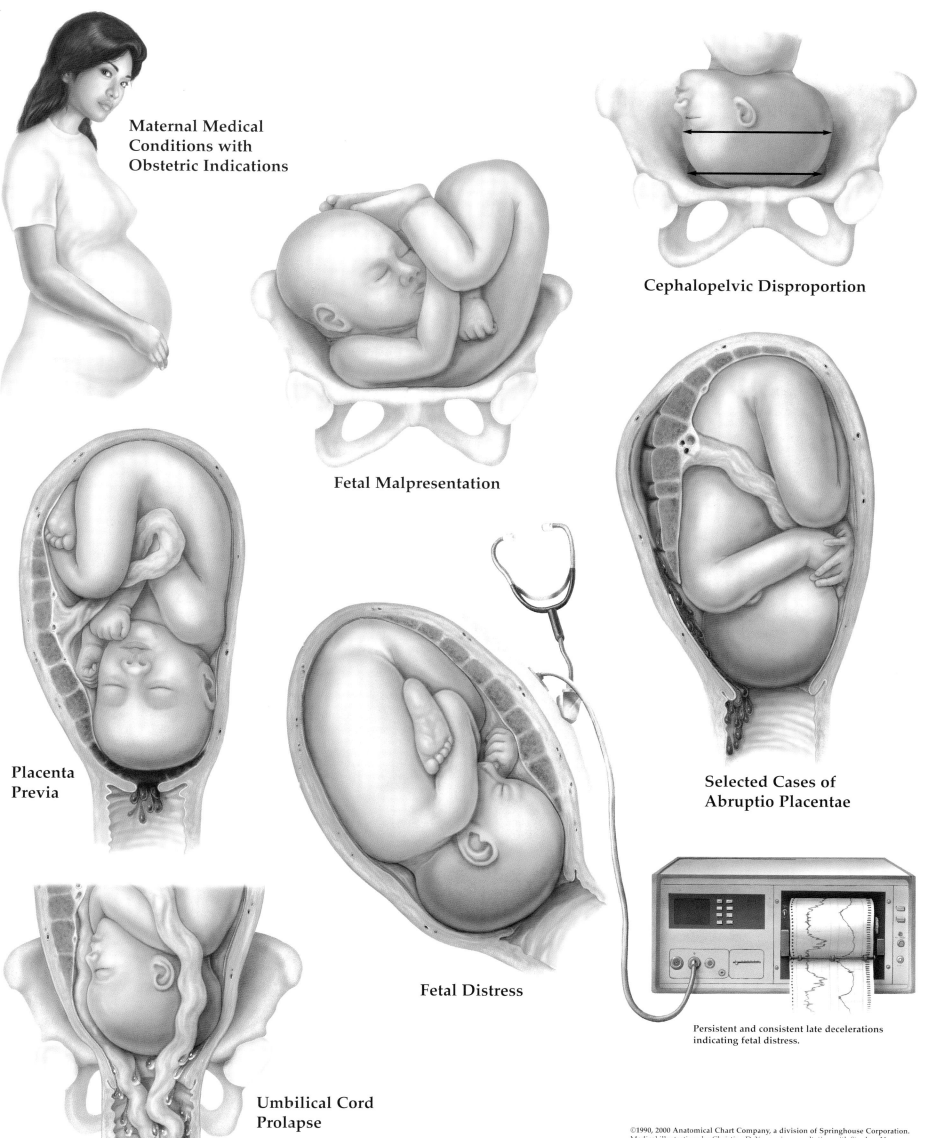

Maternal Medical Conditions with Obstetric Indications

Cephalopelvic Disproportion

Fetal Malpresentation

Placenta Previa

Selected Cases of Abruptio Placentae

Fetal Distress

Umbilical Cord Prolapse

Persistent and consistent late decelerations indicating fetal distress.

©1990, 2000 Anatomical Chart Company, a division of Springhouse Corporation. Medical illustrations by Christine D. Young, in consultation with Stephen H. Cruikshank, M.D., chief, Department of Obstetrics and Gynecology, Hennepin County Medical Center; associate professor, University of Minnesota Medical School.

9985

11

UNDERSTANDING CHOLESTEROL

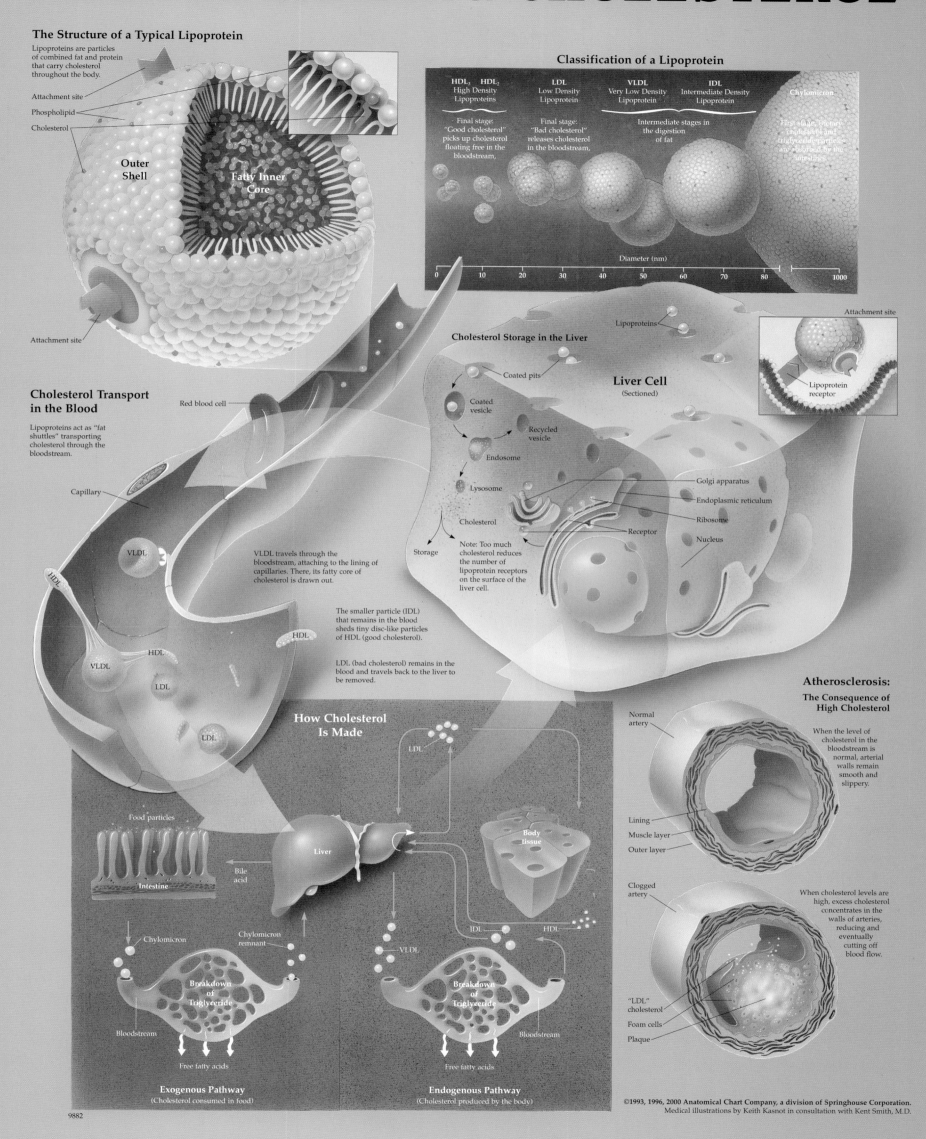

The Structure of a Typical Lipoprotein

Lipoproteins are particles of combined fat and protein that carry cholesterol throughout the body.

Attachment site
Phospholipid
Cholesterol

Outer Shell

Fatty Inner Core

Attachment site

Classification of a Lipoprotein

| HDL₁ HDL₂ High Density Lipoproteins | LDL Low Density Lipoprotein | VLDL Very Low Density Lipoprotein | IDL Intermediate Density Lipoprotein | Chylomicron |

Final stage: "Good cholesterol" picks up cholesterol floating free in the bloodstream.

Final stage: "Bad cholesterol" releases cholesterol in the bloodstream.

Intermediate stages in the digestion of fat

First stage: Dietary cholesterol and triglyceride particles are absorbed by the intestines.

Diameter (nm)

0   10   20   30   40   50   60   70   80   1000

Cholesterol Transport in the Blood

Lipoproteins act as "fat shuttles" transporting cholesterol through the bloodstream.

Red blood cell

Capillary

VLDL

HDL

HDL

HDL

VLDL

LDL

LDL

VLDL travels through the bloodstream, attaching to the lining of capillaries. There, its fatty core of cholesterol is drawn out.

The smaller particle (IDL) that remains in the blood sheds tiny disc-like particles of HDL (good cholesterol).

LDL (bad cholesterol) remains in the blood and travels back to the liver to be removed.

Cholesterol Storage in the Liver

Lipoproteins

Coated pits

Coated vesicle

Recycled vesicle

Endosome

Lysosome

Cholesterol

Storage

Liver Cell (Sectioned)

Golgi apparatus
Endoplasmic reticulum
Ribosome
Receptor
Nucleus

Note: Too much cholesterol reduces the number of lipoprotein receptors on the surface of the liver cell.

Attachment site

Lipoprotein receptor

How Cholesterol Is Made

LDL

Food particles

Liver

Bile acid

Intestine

Body tissue

IDL   HDL

Chylomicron

Chylomicron remnant

VLDL

Breakdown of Triglyceride

Breakdown of Triglyceride

Bloodstream

Bloodstream

Free fatty acids

Free fatty acids

Exogenous Pathway
(Cholesterol consumed in food)

Endogenous Pathway
(Cholesterol produced by the body)

Atherosclerosis:

The Consequence of High Cholesterol

Normal artery

When the level of cholesterol in the bloodstream is normal, arterial walls remain smooth and slippery.

Lining
Muscle layer
Outer layer

Clogged artery

When cholesterol levels are high, excess cholesterol concentrates in the walls of arteries, reducing and eventually cutting off blood flow.

"LDL" cholesterol
Foam cells
Plaque

9882

UNDERSTANDING THE COMMON COLD

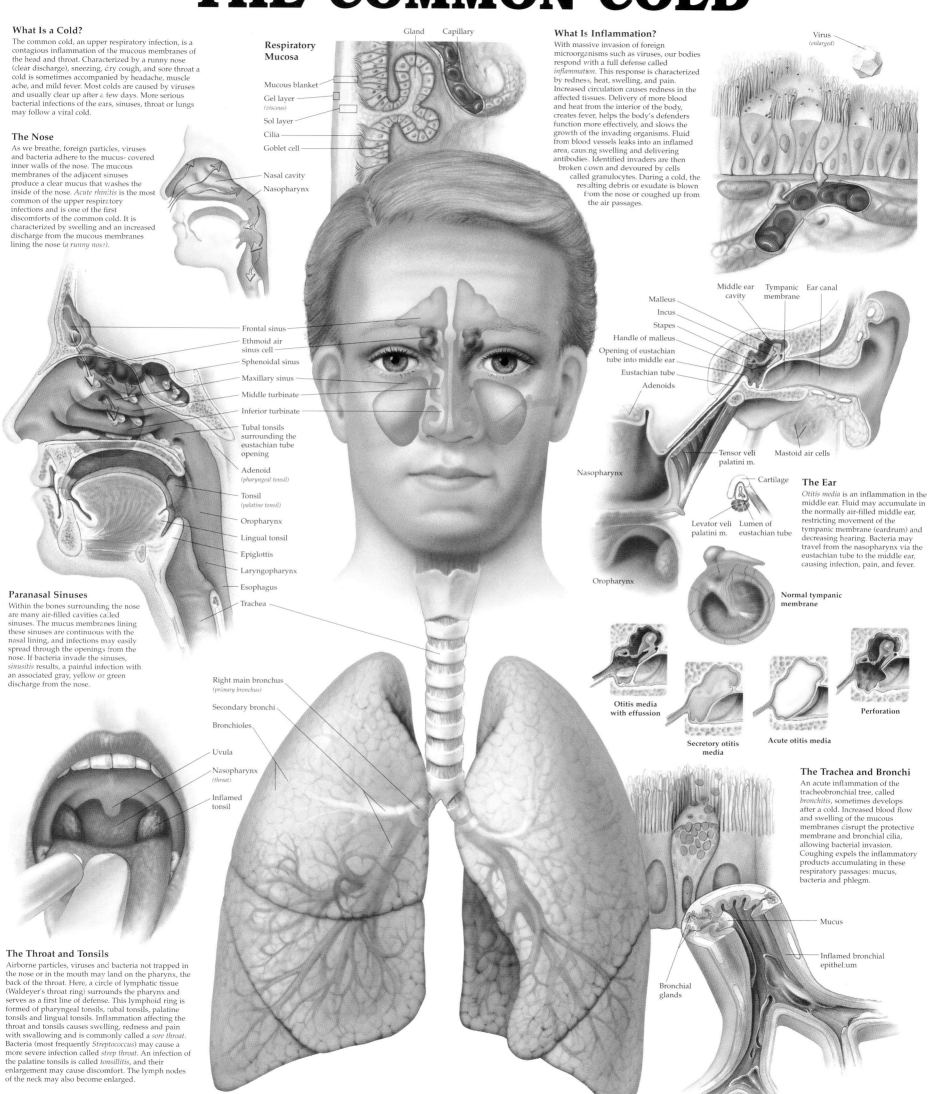

What Is a Cold?

The common cold, an upper respiratory infection, is a contagious inflammation of the mucous membranes of the head and throat. Characterized by a runny nose (clear discharge), sneezing, dry cough, and sore throat a cold is sometimes accompanied by headache, muscle ache, and mild fever. Most colds are caused by viruses and usually clear up after a few days. More serious bacterial infections of the ears, sinuses, throat or lungs may follow a viral cold.

The Nose

As we breathe, foreign particles, viruses and bacteria adhere to the mucus- covered inner walls of the nose. The mucous membranes of the adjacent sinuses produce a clear mucus that washes the inside of the nose. *Acute rhinitis* is the most common of the upper respiratory infections and is one of the first discomforts of the common cold. It is characterized by swelling and an increased discharge from the mucous membranes lining the nose (*a runny nose*).

Paranasal Sinuses

Within the bones surrounding the nose are many air-filled cavities called sinuses. The mucus membranes lining these sinuses are continuous with the nasal lining, and infections may easily spread through the openings from the nose. If bacteria invade the sinuses, *sinusitis* results, a painful infection with an associated gray, yellow or green discharge from the nose.

The Throat and Tonsils

Airborne particles, viruses and bacteria not trapped in the nose or in the mouth may land on the pharynx, the back of the throat. Here, a circle of lymphatic tissue (Waldeyer's throat ring) surrounds the pharynx and serves as a first line of defense. This lymphoid ring is formed of pharyngeal tonsils, tubal tonsils, palatine tonsils and lingual tonsils. Inflammation affecting the throat and tonsils causes swelling, redness and pain with swallowing and is commonly called a *sore throat*. Bacteria (most frequently *Streptococcus*) may cause a more severe infection called *strep throat*. An infection of the palatine tonsils is called *tonsillitis*, and their enlargement may cause discomfort. The lymph nodes of the neck may also become enlarged.

Respiratory Mucosa

Gland
Capillary
Mucous blanket
Gel layer *(viscous)*
Sol layer
Cilia
Goblet cell

Nasal cavity
Nasopharynx

Frontal sinus
Ethmoid air sinus cell
Sphenoidal sinus
Maxillary sinus
Middle turbinate
Inferior turbinate
Tubal tonsils surrounding the eustachian tube opening
Adenoid *(pharyngeal tonsil)*
Tonsil *(palatine tonsil)*
Oropharynx
Lingual tonsil
Epiglottis
Laryngopharynx
Esophagus
Trachea

Right main bronchus *(primary bronchus)*
Secondary bronchi
Bronchioles
Uvula
Nasopharynx *(throat)*
Inflamed tonsil

What Is Inflammation?

With massive invasion of foreign microorganisms such as viruses, our bodies respond with a full defense called *inflammation*. This response is characterized by redness, heat, swelling, and pain. Increased circulation causes redness in the affected tissues. Delivery of more blood and heat from the interior of the body, creates fever, helps the body's defenders function more effectively, and slows the growth of the invading organisms. Fluid from blood vessels leaks into an inflamed area, causing swelling and delivering antibodies. Identified invaders are then broken down and devoured by cells called granulocytes. During a cold, the resulting debris or exudate is blown from the nose or coughed up from the air passages.

Virus *(enlarged)*

Middle ear cavity
Tympanic membrane
Ear canal
Malleus
Incus
Stapes
Handle of malleus
Opening of eustachian tube into middle ear
Eustachian tube
Adenoids
Nasopharynx
Tensor veli palatini m.
Mastoid air cells
Oropharynx
Cartilage
Levator veli palatini m.
Lumen of eustachian tube

The Ear

Otitis media is an inflammation in the middle ear. Fluid may accumulate in the normally air-filled middle ear, restricting movement of the tympanic membrane (eardrum) and decreasing hearing. Bacteria may travel from the nasopharynx via the eustachian tube to the middle ear, causing infection, pain, and fever.

Normal tympanic membrane

Otitis media with effusion
Secretory otitis media
Acute otitis media
Perforation

The Trachea and Bronchi

An acute inflammation of the tracheobronchial tree, called *bronchitis*, sometimes develops after a cold. Increased blood flow and swelling of the mucous membranes disrupt the protective membrane and bronchial cilia, allowing bacterial invasion. Coughing expels the inflammatory products accumulating in these respiratory passages: mucus, bacteria and phlegm.

Mucus
Inflamed bronchial epithelium
Bronchial glands

9875

13

UNDERSTANDING DIABETES

What Is Diabetes?

Diabetes is the name for a group of chronic or lifelong diseases that affect the way the body uses food to make the energy necessary for life. Primarily, diabetes is a disruption of carbohydrate (sugar and starch) metabolism that also affects fats and proteins. There are two main forms of diabetes (Type I and Type II), as well as conditions of glucose intolerance, diabetes of pregnancy, and diabetes caused by pancreatic disorders. Regardless of your form of diabetes, metabolic control under your physician's care is essential for your good health.

Type I (Insulin-Dependent) Diabetes Mellitus

In Type I diabetes, the pancreas makes little or no insulin. Without insulin, sugar cannot enter cells to be used for energy. The body's tissues are starved and blood glucose levels grow dangerously high. It begins most often in youth, but it may also occur in older adults. Five percent to ten percent of diabetes patients have Type I diabetes and require insulin therapy as their treatment.

What Is Insulin?

Insulin is an essential hormone produced in the pancreas and released into the bloodstream. Insulin attaches itself to cells at places called insulin receptors. Once attached, insulin allows sugar or glucose from the food we eat to enter the liver, fat, and muscle cells, where it is used for energy.

Type II (Non-Insulin-Dependent) Diabetes Mellitus

In Type II diabetes, the pancreas produces some insulin, but it is either too little or is not effective. Also, insulin receptors that control the transport of sugar into cells may not work properly or are reduced in number. Type II diabetes most often develops in people over 40 years of age. A majority of newly diagnosed Type II patients are overweight but are able to control their diabetes through diet and weight loss. Some patients may require oral medications or insulin injections to achieve glucose control.

Symptoms of Diabetes

Sudden weight loss	Type I
Fatigue or tiredness	
Increased hunger	
Increased thirst	
Increased urination *(volume and frequency)*	Type I or Type II
Frequent infections *(periodontal disease, urinary tract infections, vaginitis)*	
Slow-healing cuts or sores	
Blurred vision	
Dry, itchy skin	
Numbness in feet, hands	
Impotence	
No symptoms	

Glucose Metabolism

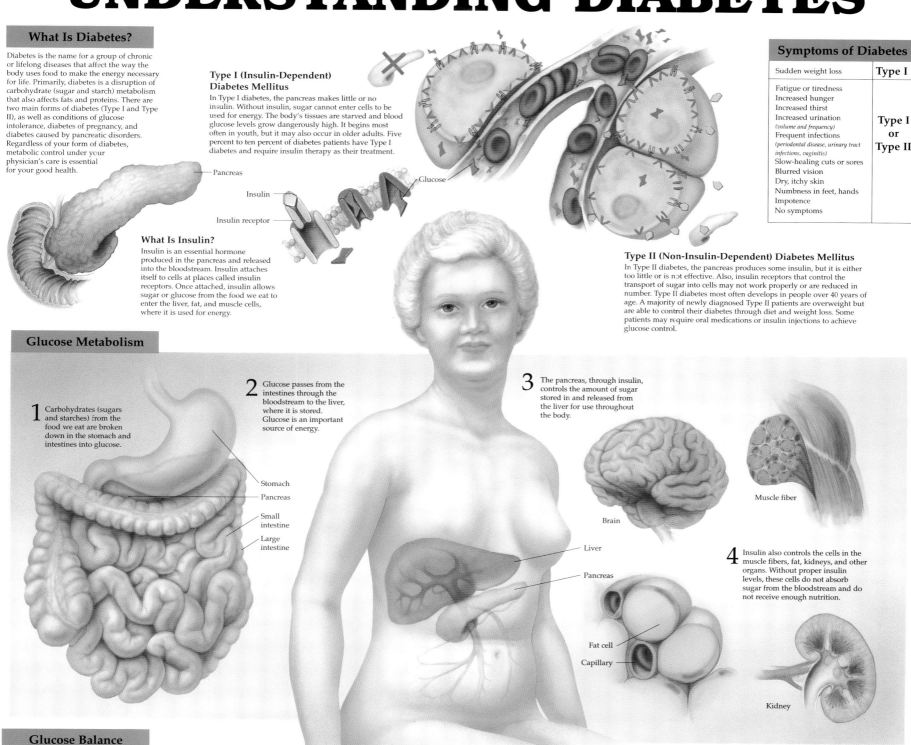

Pancreas
Insulin
Insulin receptor
Glucose

1 Carbohydrates (sugars and starches) from the food we eat are broken down in the stomach and intestines into glucose.

2 Glucose passes from the intestines through the bloodstream to the liver, where it is stored. Glucose is an important source of energy.

3 The pancreas, through insulin, controls the amount of sugar stored in and released from the liver for use throughout the body.

4 Insulin also controls the cells in the muscle fibers, fat, kidneys, and other organs. Without proper insulin levels, these cells do not absorb sugar from the bloodstream and do not receive enough nutrition.

Stomach
Pancreas
Small intestine
Large intestine
Brain
Muscle fiber
Liver
Pancreas
Fat cell
Capillary
Kidney

Glucose Balance

Precise levels of sugar or glucose are maintained in the blood, depending on the body's needs for energy. Your doctor can monitor your glucose level history with a glycosylated hemoglobin test.

Too little sugar in one's blood

Too much sugar in one's blood

Hyperglycemia	Hypoglycemia
Caused by:	
Too little insulin	Too much insulin
Overeating	Too little food
Illness or stress	Excessive exercise
Inactivity	
Symptoms:	
Fatigue	Hunger
Abdominal pain	Trembling or weakness
Weight loss	Sweating
Thirst	Confusion or irritability
Irritability	
Results in:	
Diabetic coma	**Insulin reaction**
Ketoacidosis	

Long-Term Health Problems

High plasma glucose levels caused by diabetes may damage small and large blood vessels and nerves. Diabetes may also lower the body's ability to fight infection. As a result, people with diabetes are more likely to have serious eye problems, kidney disease, heart attacks, strokes, high blood pressure, poor circulation, tingling in hands and feet, sexual problems, amputations, and infections. Good diabetes control may help prevent these problems or make them less serious.

Healthy Lifestyle Changes

Learning as much as possible about diabetes can help you effectively manage your diabetes and make healthy lifestyle changes. These changes include:

- Selecting a balanced diet high in complex carbohydrates,
- Limiting simple carbohydrates or sugars
- Decreasing dietary fat
- Timing meals carefully
- Enjoying low-impact exercises such as walking, swimming or cycling

It is very important to follow your physician's instructions and to see your team of diabetes healthcare professionals regularly. Consult them before beginning any diet and/or exercise program.

Loss of Vision **Nerve Damage** **Poor Circulation** **Heart Disease** **Kidney Failure**

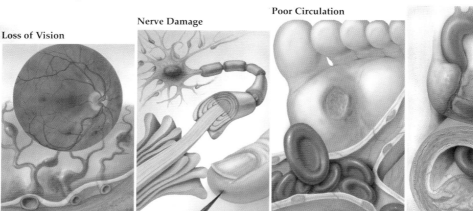

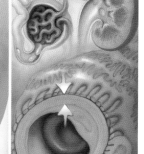

9755

14

DISEASES OF THE DIGESTIVE SYSTEM

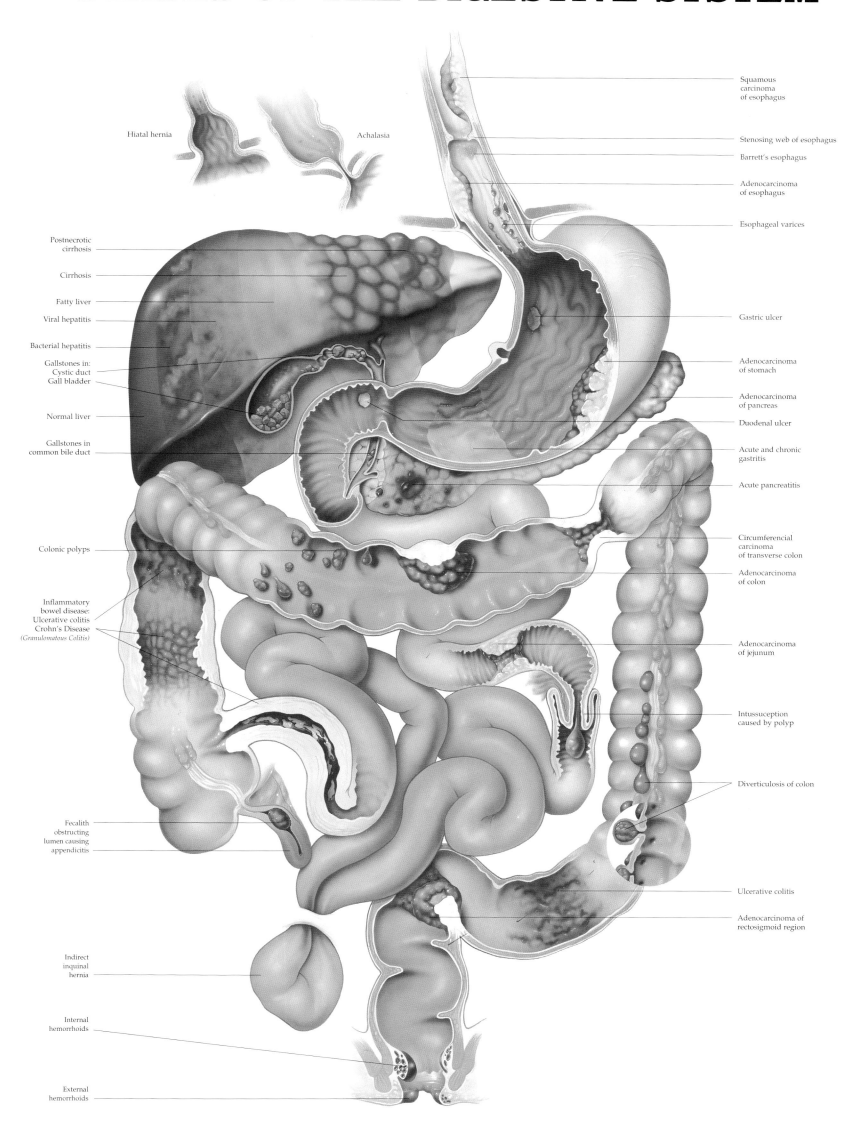

Hiatal hernia

Achalasia

Squamous carcinoma of esophagus

Stenosing web of esophagus

Barrett's esophagus

Adenocarcinoma of esophagus

Esophageal varices

Postnecrotic cirrhosis

Cirrhosis

Fatty liver

Viral hepatitis

Bacterial hepatitis

Gallstones in: Cystic duct Gall bladder

Normal liver

Gallstones in common bile duct

Gastric ulcer

Adenocarcinoma of stomach

Adenocarcinoma of pancreas

Duodenal ulcer

Acute and chronic gastritis

Acute pancreatitis

Colonic polyps

Circumferencial carcinoma of transverse colon

Adenocarcinoma of colon

Inflammatory bowel disease: Ulcerative colitis Crohn's Disease (Granulomatous Colitis)

Adenocarcinoma of jejunum

Intussuception caused by polyp

Fecalith obstructing lumen causing appendicitis

Diverticulosis of colon

Indirect inquinal hernia

Ulcerative colitis

Adenocarcinoma of rectosigmoid region

Internal hemorrhoids

External hemorrhoids

UNDERSTANDING EPILEPSY

What Is Epilepsy?

Epilepsy is a common neurological condition that affects millions of people throughout the world. The term "epilepsy" is a general name that refers to many different disorders in which people tend to experience seizures. Other conditions, such as high fever, the use of or withdrawal from drugs or alcohol, or a blow to the head, can cause an isolated seizure. Only those people who have had two or more seizures are diagnosed as having epilepsy.

What Causes Epilepsy?

Many cases of epilepsy are said to be symptomatic. This means they are the result of other conditions such as a birth injury, head injury, stroke, brain tumor, infection, or congenital abnormality. Genetic factors may also play a role in the cause of epilepsy. Some cases of epilepsy, however, remain idiopathic, meaning they develop for reasons which we presently cannot determine.

How the Brain Works

Although it appears to be solid, the brain is made up of billions of cells, including a network of cells called neurons. These neurons branch out, much like branches on a tree. This neural network enables communication within the brain and between the brain and the rest of the body.

Neurons

When a neuron "fires" it sends small electrical impulses along its branches toward surrounding cells. At the end of each branch is a small gap or synapse, which the impulse must overcome in order to continue its journey.

When an impulse reaches the end of a branch, chemicals called neurotransmitters are released to flood the synapse. Some are excitatory, stimulating the neighboring cell to fire. Others are inhibitory, making the next cell less likely to fire.

The brain's ability to turn electrical impulses "on" and "off" allows it to control messages and work effectively. Since normal behavior is the result of many neurons working together, a fine balance of excitatory and inhibitory factors is needed to insure that the correct neurons fire at the appropriate times. In people with epilepsy, however, this fine balance is upset, making the brain unable to limit the spread of electrical activity. When too many neurons fire at once, an electrical storm is created within the brain.

Vesicles release neurotransmitters, which flood the synapse.

Frontal
motor control, some aspects of personality

Parietal
sensation, some aspects of language

Occipital
vision

Temporal
speech, hearing

The brain is divided into two hemispheres. The right half controls the left side of the body and the left half controls the right side of the body. Each hemisphere is divided into four lobes. Within the lobes there are even smaller areas, each associated with specific functions.

What Is a Seizure?

A seizure is an excessive discharge of electrical activity within the brain, which leads to a change in movement, sensation, experience, or consciousness. There are many types of seizures. The effects they have on the body vary greatly, depending on where in the brain the seizure starts and where it spreads.

Phases of a Seizure

Aura: an unusual sensation or peculiar feeling often felt prior to a more widespread seizure. Can also be called a simple partial seizure.

Ictus: the whole seizure, including the aura.

Post-ictus: time after a seizure; may experience muscle weakness or deep sleep.

Seizures Can Cause:

- A twitching muscle
- Convulsive movements
- A tingling sensation
- Sweating
- The perception of an unusual smell or taste
- Hallucinations
- Fear or anxiety
- Changes in awareness
- Loss of consciousness
- Other changes

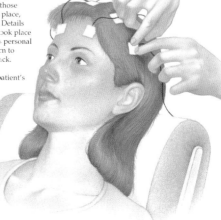

This illustration shows a seizure originating in the left motor strip, affecting movement of the fingers, hand, and arm.

If Someone Has a Seizure

Although big seizures may be frightening to witness, they are usually not medical emergencies. In most cases the seizure itself is not harmful to the individual who is having it and therefore should be allowed to run its course. An ambulance is usually not necessary unless the seizure lasts longer than ten minutes, there are multiple, repeated seizures, or the person is injured, diabetic or pregnant. There is nothing family or friends can do to stop a seizure, but certain steps can be taken to prevent further injury.

You Should:

- Stay calm
- Help the person lie down and roll onto one side to prevent choking
- Loosen tight, restrictive clothing and remove eyeglasses
- Protect the person's head with a soft object such as a pillow or jacket
- Gently guide a conscious but confused person away from hazards
- Remain with the person until s/he is awake and alert
- Be comforting and reassuring

You Should Not:

- Put anything into the person's mouth
- Try to restrain the person

Generalized Seizures

These seizures affect both hemispheres of the brain at the same time. Abnormal activity is not focused in one specific area and there generally is no aura at the start.

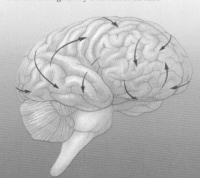

Partial Seizures

These seizures begin in a part of one hemisphere, generally in the temporal or frontal lobe. The two types of partial seizures, called simple and complex, are based on whether a person remains fully conscious during a seizure.

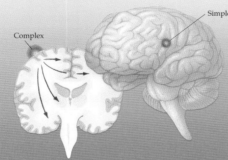

Simple

Complex

Diagnosing Epilepsy

There is no single test for epilepsy. The doctor will make a diagnosis based on a description of past seizures. Since those who have had a seizure are often unaware of what took place, the doctor may rely on others who witnessed the event. Details about how the patient felt before the attack and how it took place are very useful. The doctor will also review the patient's personal and family medical history, and will give a physical exam to check for other conditions that may have caused the attack.

There are tests designed to gather information about a patient's condition. The most commonly used test is an electroencephalogram (EEG). An EEG involves attaching a series of metal discs called electrodes to the patient's head to measure the brain's electrical activity. Most types of seizures are detectable with the EEG, but some abnormal activity may affect too small an area on the brain's surface or be located too deep to be detected. Other tests such as computed tomography (CT) and magnetic resonance imaging (MRI) can provide additional information about the brain. A doctor may order these tests to look for causes of the attack, such as a tumor, congenital malformation, or other changes in the brain.

Main Forms of Generalized Seizures

Absence seizures:

- **Typical** absence seizures (formerly called "petit mal") – result in brief episodes of impaired awareness. There also may be small motor movements, changes in muscle tone, or automatic behaviors.
- **Atonic** seizures – associated with a sudden loss of muscle tone in a limb or throughout the entire body. The person having the seizure will often drop things or fall to the ground.
- **Myoclonic** seizures – sudden shock-like jolt to one or more muscles which increases muscle tone and causes movement. These sudden jerks are like those that occur in healthy people as they fall asleep.
- **Tonic-clonic** seizures (formerly called "grand mal") – begin with simultaneous loss of consciousness and the tonic phase (stiffening of the body). The person falls to the ground and often emits a loud cry as the chest muscles stiffen. Next comes the clonic phase, during which the muscles rhythmically jerk.

Main Forms of Partial Seizures

Simple partial seizures (sometimes called "auras"):

Seizure activity is focused in a specific area of the brain. A person remains alert and afterward is able to remember what happened. An aura or simple partial seizure may constitute the entire seizure or may precede a complex partial or generalized seizure. Symptoms vary depending on the area of the brain involved.

- Motor seizures cause a change in muscle activity and may involve jerking or stiffening of a part of the body.
- Sensory seizures may cause abnormal function in any of the five senses.
- Autonomic seizures affect involuntary functions and may cause a rapid heartbeat or breathing rate, sweating, or an unpleasant sensation in the abdomen, chest, throat or head.
- Psychic seizures may affect perception and memory or stimulate emotions such as fear.

Complex partial seizures:

Seizure is accompanied by impaired consciousness and recall. May also involve staring, automatic behaviors such as lip smacking, chewing, fumbling, picking, walking, grunting, repetition of words or phrases, or other symptoms and signs.

9867

i

DISORDERS OF THE EYE

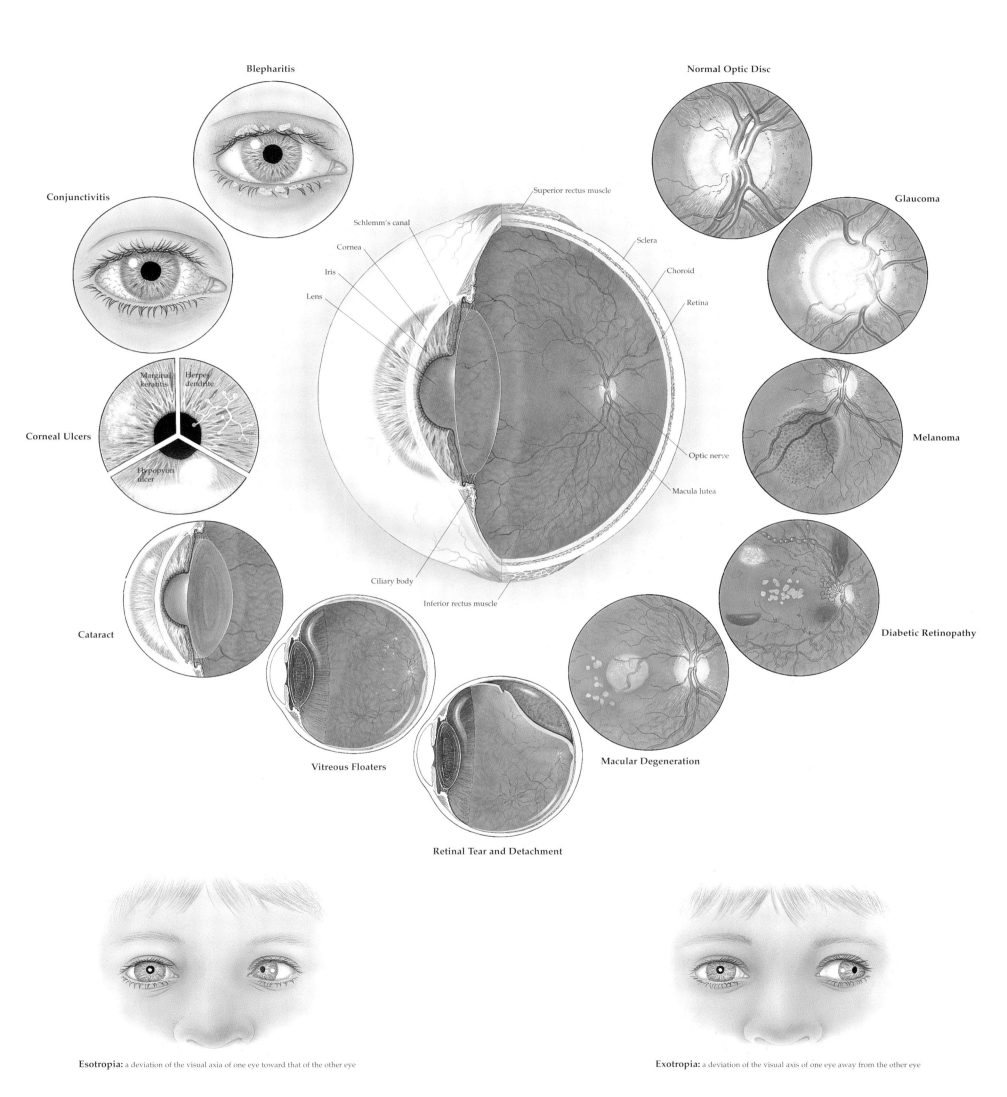

Blepharitis

Conjunctivitis

Corneal Ulcers

Marginal keratitis

Herpes dendrite

Hypopyon ulcer

Cataract

Vitreous Floaters

Retinal Tear and Detachment

Superior rectus muscle

Schlemm's canal

Cornea

Iris

Lens

Sclera

Choroid

Retina

Optic nerve

Macula lutea

Ciliary body

Inferior rectus muscle

Normal Optic Disc

Glaucoma

Melanoma

Diabetic Retinopathy

Macular Degeneration

Esotropia: a deviation of the visual axis of one eye toward that of the other eye

Exotropia: a deviation of the visual axis of one eye away from the other eye

9695

©1992, 2000 Anatomical Chart Company, a division of Springhouse Corporation.
Medical illustrations by Linda Warren, in consultation with David B. Pugh, M.D.

HEART DISEASE

Progression of Heart Disease in Atherosclerosis

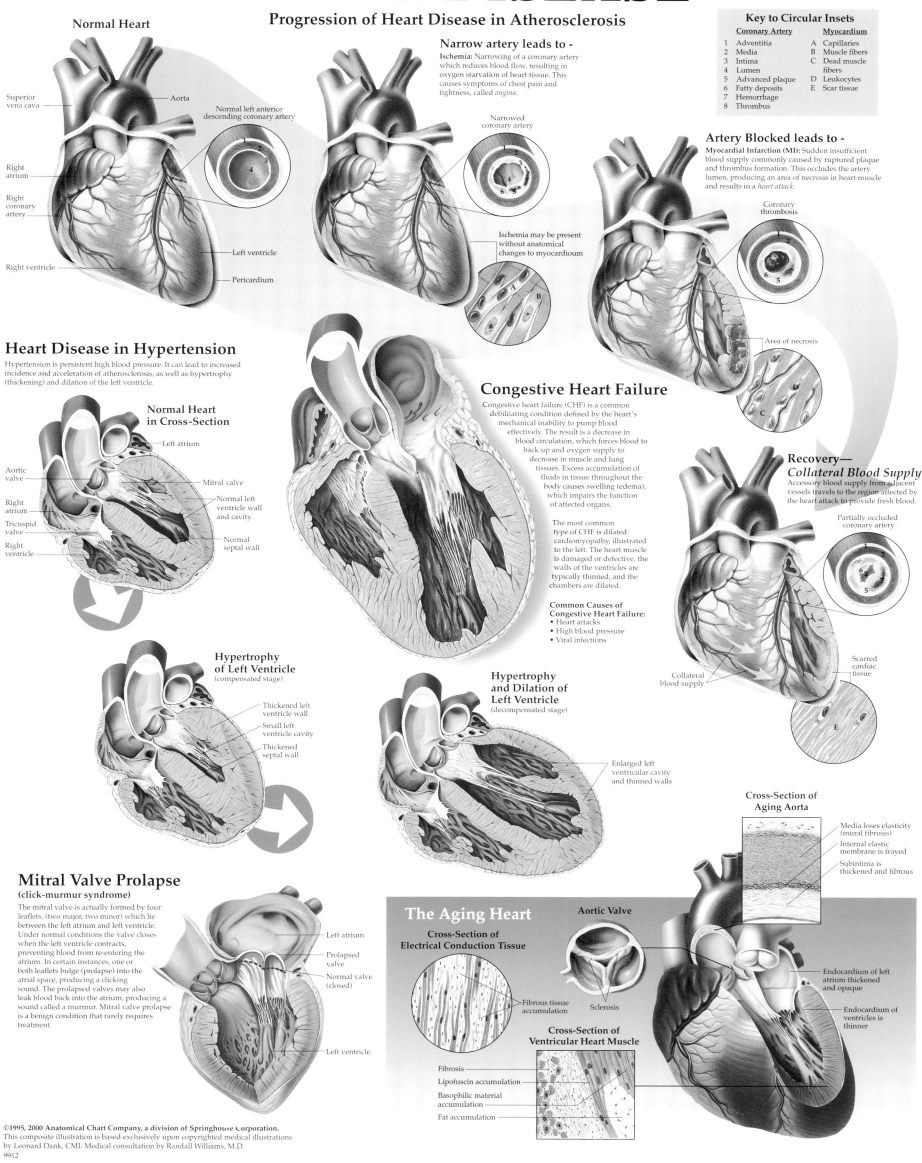

Normal Heart

- Superior vena cava
- Aorta
- Right atrium
- Right coronary artery
- Right ventricle
- Left ventricle
- Pericardium
- Normal left anterior descending coronary artery

Narrow artery leads to -

Ischemia: Narrowing of a coronary artery which reduces blood flow, resulting in oxygen starvation of heart tissue. This causes symptoms of chest pain and tightness, called *angina*.

Narrowed coronary artery

Ischemia may be present without anatomical changes to myocardium

Artery Blocked leads to -

Myocardial Infarction (MI): Sudden insufficient blood supply commonly caused by ruptured plaque and thrombus formation. This occludes the artery lumen, producing an area of necrosis in heart muscle and results in a *heart attack*.

Coronary thrombosis

Area of necrosis

Key to Circular Insets

Coronary Artery		Myocardium	
1	Adventitia	A	Capillaries
2	Media	B	Muscle fibers
3	Intima	C	Dead muscle fibers
4	Lumen		
5	Advanced plaque	D	Leukocytes
6	Fatty deposits	E	Scar tissue
7	Hemorrhage		
8	Thrombus		

Heart Disease in Hypertension

Hypertension is persistent high blood pressure. It can lead to increased incidence and acceleration of atherosclerosis, as well as hypertrophy (thickening) and dilation of the left ventricle.

Normal Heart in Cross-Section

- Left atrium
- Aortic valve
- Mitral valve
- Right atrium
- Normal left ventricle wall and cavity
- Tricuspid valve
- Right ventricle
- Normal septal wall

Hypertrophy of Left Ventricle
(compensated stage)

- Thickened left ventricle wall
- Small left ventricle cavity
- Thickened septal wall

Hypertrophy and Dilation of Left Ventricle
(decompensated stage)

- Enlarged left ventricular cavity and thinned walls

Congestive Heart Failure

Congestive heart failure (CHF) is a common debilitating condition defined by the heart's mechanical inability to pump blood effectively. The result is a decrease in blood circulation, which forces blood to back up and oxygen supply to decrease in muscle and lung tissues. Excess accumulation of fluids in tissue throughout the body causes swelling (edema), which impairs the function of affected organs.

The most common type of CHF is dilated cardiomyopathy, illustrated to the left. The heart muscle is damaged or defective, the walls of the ventricles are typically thinned, and the chambers are dilated.

Common Causes of Congestive Heart Failure:
- Heart attacks
- High blood pressure
- Viral infections

Recovery— Collateral Blood Supply

Accessory blood supply from adjacent vessels travels to the region affected by the heart attack to provide fresh blood.

- Partially occluded coronary artery
- Collateral blood supply
- Scarred cardiac tissue

Mitral Valve Prolapse
(click-murmur syndrome)

The mitral valve is actually formed by four leaflets, (two major, two minor) which lie between the left atrium and left ventricle. Under normal conditions the valve closes when the left ventricle contracts, preventing blood from re-entering the atrium. In certain instances, one or both leaflets bulge (prolapse) into the atrial space, producing a clicking sound. The prolapsed valves may also leak blood back into the atrium, producing a sound called a murmur. Mitral valve prolapse is a benign condition that rarely requires treatment.

- Left atrium
- Prolapsed valve
- Normal valve (closed)
- Left ventricle

Cross-Section of Aging Aorta

- Media loses elasticity (mural fibrosis)
- Internal elastic membrane is frayed
- Subintima is thickened and fibrous

The Aging Heart

Aortic Valve
- Sclerosis

Cross-Section of Electrical Conduction Tissue
- Fibrous tissue accumulation

Cross-Section of Ventricular Heart Muscle
- Fibrosis
- Lipofuscin accumulation
- Basophilic material accumulation
- Fat accumulation

- Endocardium of left atrium thickened and opaque
- Endocardium of ventricles is thinner

HIP AND KNEE INFLAMMATIONS

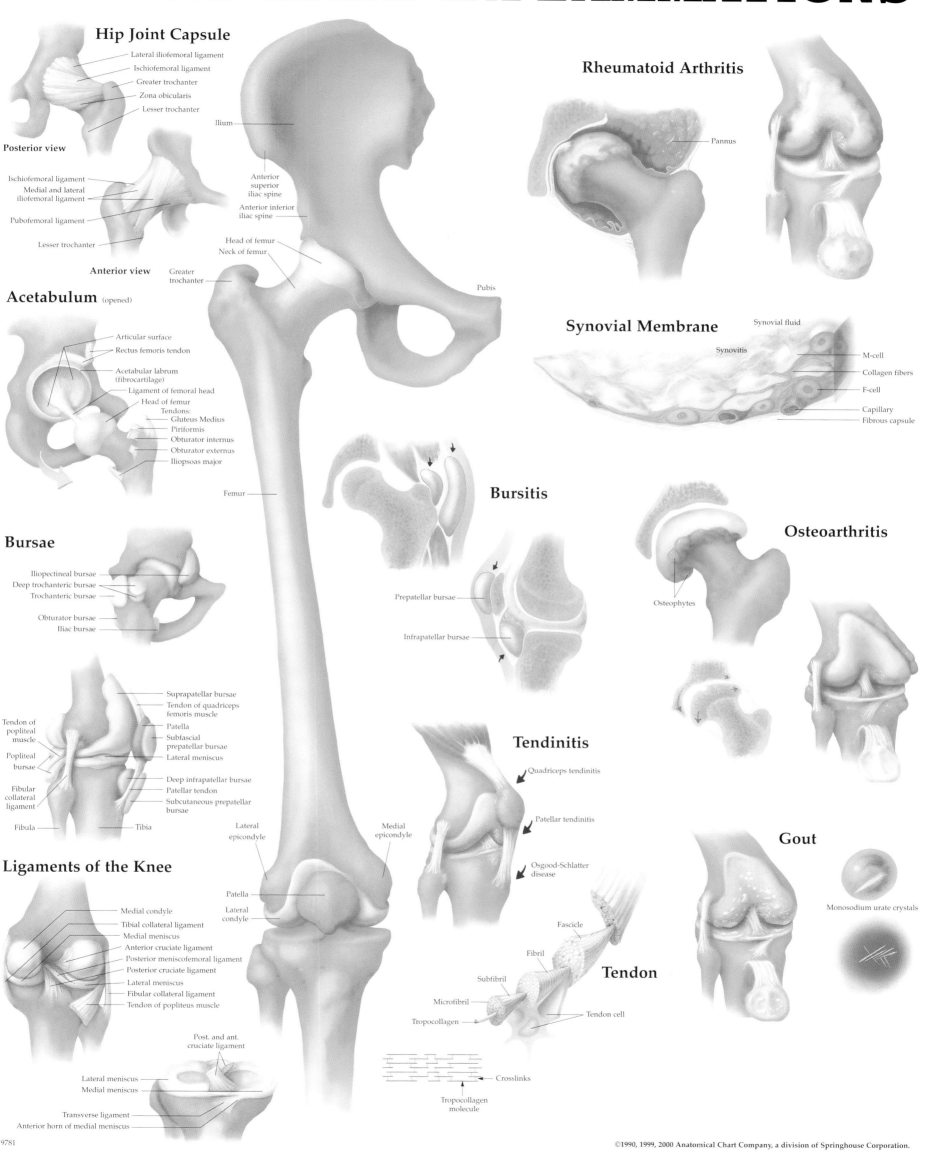

Hip Joint Capsule

- Lateral iliofemoral ligament
- Ischiofemoral ligament
- Greater trochanter
- Zona obicularis
- Lesser trochanter

Posterior view

- Ischiofemoral ligament
- Medial and lateral iliofemoral ligament
- Pubofemoral ligament
- Lesser trochanter

Anterior view

Acetabulum (opened)

- Articular surface
- Rectus femoris tendon
- Acetabular labrum (fibrocartilage)
- Ligament of femoral head
- Head of femur
- Tendons:
  - Gluteus Medius
  - Piriformis
  - Obturator internus
  - Obturator externus
  - Iliopsoas major

Bursae

- Iliopectineal bursae
- Deep trochanteric bursae
- Trochanteric bursae
- Obturator bursae
- Iliac bursae

- Suprapatellar bursae
- Tendon of quadriceps femoris muscle
- Patella
- Subfascial prepatellar bursae
- Lateral meniscus
- Tendon of popliteal muscle
- Popliteal bursae
- Deep infrapatellar bursae
- Patellar tendon
- Subcutaneous prepatellar bursae
- Fibular collateral ligament
- Fibula
- Tibia

Ligaments of the Knee

- Medial condyle
- Tibial collateral ligament
- Medial meniscus
- Anterior cruciate ligament
- Posterior meniscofemoral ligament
- Posterior cruciate ligament
- Lateral meniscus
- Fibular collateral ligament
- Tendon of popliteus muscle

- Post. and ant. cruciate ligament
- Lateral meniscus
- Medial meniscus
- Transverse ligament
- Anterior horn of medial meniscus

Ilium

- Anterior superior iliac spine
- Anterior inferior iliac spine
- Head of femur
- Neck of femur
- Greater trochanter
- Pubis

- Femur

- Lateral epicondyle
- Medial epicondyle
- Patella
- Lateral condyle

Rheumatoid Arthritis

- Pannus

Synovial Membrane

- Synovial fluid
- Synovitis
- M-cell
- Collagen fibers
- F-cell
- Capillary
- Fibrous capsule

Bursitis

- Prepatellar bursae
- Infrapatellar bursae

Osteoarthritis

- Osteophytes

Tendinitis

- Quadriceps tendinitis
- Patellar tendinitis
- Osgood-Schlatter disease

Tendon

- Fascicle
- Fibril
- Subfibril
- Microfibril
- Tropocollagen
- Tendon cell

- Crosslinks
- Tropocollagen molecule

Gout

- Monosodium urate crystals

UNDERSTANDING HIV & AIDS

What Is AIDS?
Acquired immunodeficiency syndrome, or AIDS is a devastating condition that develops after the immune system has been severely weakened and can no longer defend the body from certain infections. As AIDS progresses, the body is overwhelmed with life-threatening illnesses and diseases.

What Is HIV?
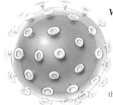

HIV is the virus that causes AIDS. It stands for human immunodeficiency virus and is referred to as the "AIDS virus." HIV destroys immune cells called T-cells, which are vital to the body for protection against infection and diseases, including cancer. AIDS results when HIV has severely reduced the number of T-cells.

HIV (AIDS virus)

Who Develops AIDS?
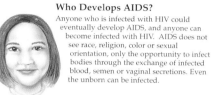

Anyone who is infected with HIV could eventually develop AIDS, and anyone can become infected with HIV. AIDS does not see race, religion, color or sexual orientation, only the opportunity to infect bodies through the exchange of infected blood, semen or vaginal secretions. Even the unborn can be infected.

How Is HIV Transmitted?
HIV lives in white blood cells called T-cells, which are found in blood, semen, breast milk and vaginal secretions, including menstrual blood. HIV can be transmitted when there is contact with infected fluids. The most common ways people become infected are through sexual activity, sharing contaminated hypodermic needles, and transmission from mother to fetus during pregnancy, birth or breast feeding.

Sexual Activity

Sexual activity is the most common way HIV is spread, especially without the use of a latex condom and spermicide. Contact with infected blood, semen or vaginal secretions can lead to the transmission of HIV as well as transmission through oral sex.

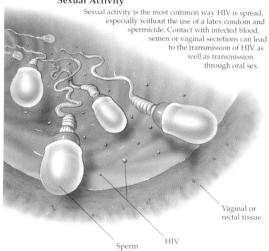

Vaginal or rectal tissue

Sperm — HIV

Injecting Drugs
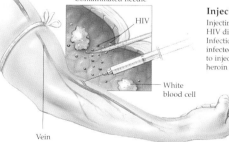

Contaminated needle
HIV
White blood cell
Vein

Injecting drugs can transmit HIV directly into the body. Infection occurs while sharing infected needles and syringes to inject drugs such as steroids, heroin and cocaine.

HIV Antibody Test
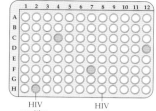

HIV antibody testing identifies HIV infection by detecting HIV antibodies in the blood. The HIV antibodies are produced in response to the presence of the virus and can be detected in the blood 4 to 12 weeks after infection. An HIV-negative result means no antibodies were found in the blood; HIV-positive means antibodies are present. A positive result is always confirmed by a second test using a different method. Other than a positive AIDS antibody test, there are often no signs of infection for years, which is why it is important to be tested if you are engaged in high-risk behavior. For testing locations contact your physician or call the National HIV/AIDS hotline.

Preliminary HIV antibody test results
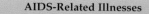

HIV positive   HIV negative

Each circle represents one person

HIV Positive
A positive HIV test means you have been infected with HIV for life and are able to infect others. Inform those with whom you have engaged in sexual activity or shared needles. Stay as healthy as possible, because even a cold or the flu can help the HIV virus weaken the immune system. Not all people with HIV develop AIDS; but most do. Take added precautions during sexual activity and drug use to prevent the spread of HIV.

Symptoms of HIV Infection

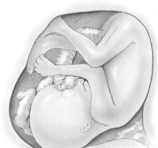

Vein — HIV
White blood cell
HIV antibodies

Memory loss, disorientation, inability to think clearly

Persistent headaches

High fever

White patches on tongue

Swollen lymph nodes in neck, armpits and groin

Heavy night sweats

Loss of appetite

Severe weight loss

Chronic diarrhea

Fatigue & muscle weakness

Stages of HIV Infection

1. Acute Infection
Occurs about one to two weeks after initial infection. During this stage the HIV virus undergoes massive replication.

2. Asymptomatic HIV
During this stage chronic signs or symptoms are not displayed. T-cell count may be used to monitor progression of the disease. With the patient's own individual resistance and drug therapy this stage can last for 10 to 12 years.

3. Symptomatic HIV
There are two phases within this stage: Early and Late. Some symptoms of the Early phase include fever, candida albicans, herpes and night sweats.

When the T-cell count falls below 200 cells per microliter, it is considered the late phase. During this phase diseases and disorders can include gastric ulcers, esophagitis, hepatitis, pancreatitis, herpes zoster, dermatitis, nausea, severe weight loss, and chronic diarrhea. Usually at least one opportunistic disease develops.

4. Advanced HIV
A T-cell count of less than 59 cells per microliter marks this stage. Symptoms include seizures, confusion, incontinence, blindness and coma. With the onset of Advanced HIV, the mortality rate increases.

AIDS-Related Illnesses

Opportunistic Infections (OIs)
OIs only occur when the immune system is severely damaged. These infections cause life-threatening illnesses in people with AIDS.

A. Cryptococcal meningitis:
Inflammation of tissue in and around the brain and central nervous system

B. Toxoplasmosis encephalitis:
The most common OI to attack the central nervous system

C. Cytomegalovirus (CMV) retinitis:
Leads to blindness

D. Herpes simplex virus (HSV):
Sores that occur around the mouth and genitals

E. Oral candidiasis (thrush):
White fungal growth that coats the tongue and mouth

F. Candida esophagitis:
Painful ulceration of the esophagus

G. Pneumocystis carinii pneumonia (PCP):
Causes fever, cough and shortness of breath

H. Pulmonary Tuberculosis:
Produces cough, sputum and difficult breathing

Cancer
Certain cancers also develop in people with AIDS. Two common AIDS related cancers are Kaposi's sarcoma (I) and non-Hodgkin's lymphoma. Kaposi's sarcoma first appears as purplish-brown lesions on the skin.

J. Cryptosporidiosis:
Major symptoms are severe diarrhea and weight loss.

> **National HIV/AIDS Hotline**
> **1-800-342-AIDS**
> En Español
> **1-800-344-SIDA**
> Hotline for the Hearing Impaired
> **1-800-AIDS-TTY**

Pregnancy
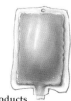

Infected body fluids from the mother are passed to her infant during pregnancy, delivery and breastfeeding. Babies born to infected mothers have a 15% to 25% chance of becoming infected.

Preventing HIV Infection
You can greatly reduce or even eliminate the risk of catching HIV. Get the information you need from your health care provider, and take these precautions:

Sex: The best protection is to delay having sex until you have established a long-term, mutually monogamous relationship with an uninfected person. Ask your partner to take the HIV antibody test before initiating a sexual relationship. Using a latex condom with a spermicide during sex will greatly reduce your chances of contracting the HIV but *will not* provide 100% protection.

Health: Stay as healthy as possible and free of sexually transmitted diseases (STDs). STD's can create open sores and inflammation on the skin and around and inside the mouth, genital and anal areas, which provide a direct route of entry for the HIV virus.

Drugs: Not using drugs and not having sex with intravenous drug users can reduce the risk of HIV infection. If injecting drugs, *never* share needles. Obtain sterile needles from a pharmacy or through a needle exchange program. To decontaminate needles and syringes, flush them three or four times with chlorine bleach and repeat with tap water. This reduces, but does not eliminate, the risk of HIV infection.

Pregnancy: An HIV test should be taken before becoming pregnant if you have engaged in high-risk behavior. The best protection for the infant is if the mother has tested HIV-negative before, during and after pregnancy and breast feeding.

Treatment
Currently, AIDS is not curable. Early detection and treatment of HIV and AIDS can increase a patient's life expectancy. There are no vaccines available to date, but medications are available to slow the progression of HIV and development of AIDS. Other medications are available to protect against and treat the variety of illnesses that may develop. Consult with a physician that specializes in caring for HIV-infected individuals. It is critical that any prescribed medication be taken as directed.

How HIV Is NOT Spread
Although HIV can be found in saliva and tears, transmission is unlikely via these liquids HIV is not spread by coughing, sneezing, crying or sweating on someone. One cannot be infected from toilets, locker rooms, showers, towels, telephones, public areas, silverware, drinking glasses, clothing, bed linen, kissing, hugging, touching or casual contact.

Blood and Blood Products
Infected blood is where HIV is found in the highest concentrations. Since 1985 the HIV antibody test has been used to screen blood donations for the virus. Now it is rare to become infected by receiving blood or blood products through transfusion. Donating blood carries no risk.

Risks for Becoming Infected with HIV

HIGH RISK	MEDIUM RISK	LOW RISK
• Anal, vaginal or oral sex without a condom	• Anal, vaginal or oral sex with a condom	• Intimate touching
• Sharing needles and syringes (not cleaned with chlorine bleach)	• Sharing needles and syringes (cleaned with chlorine bleach)	• Blood transfusion (after 1985)
• Sex with injecting-drug users or other high risk individuals	• Infected body fluids contacting open wounds and sores	• Organ transplant
• Multiple sex partners		• Deep kissing

9760

THE HUMAN SPINE—DISORDERS

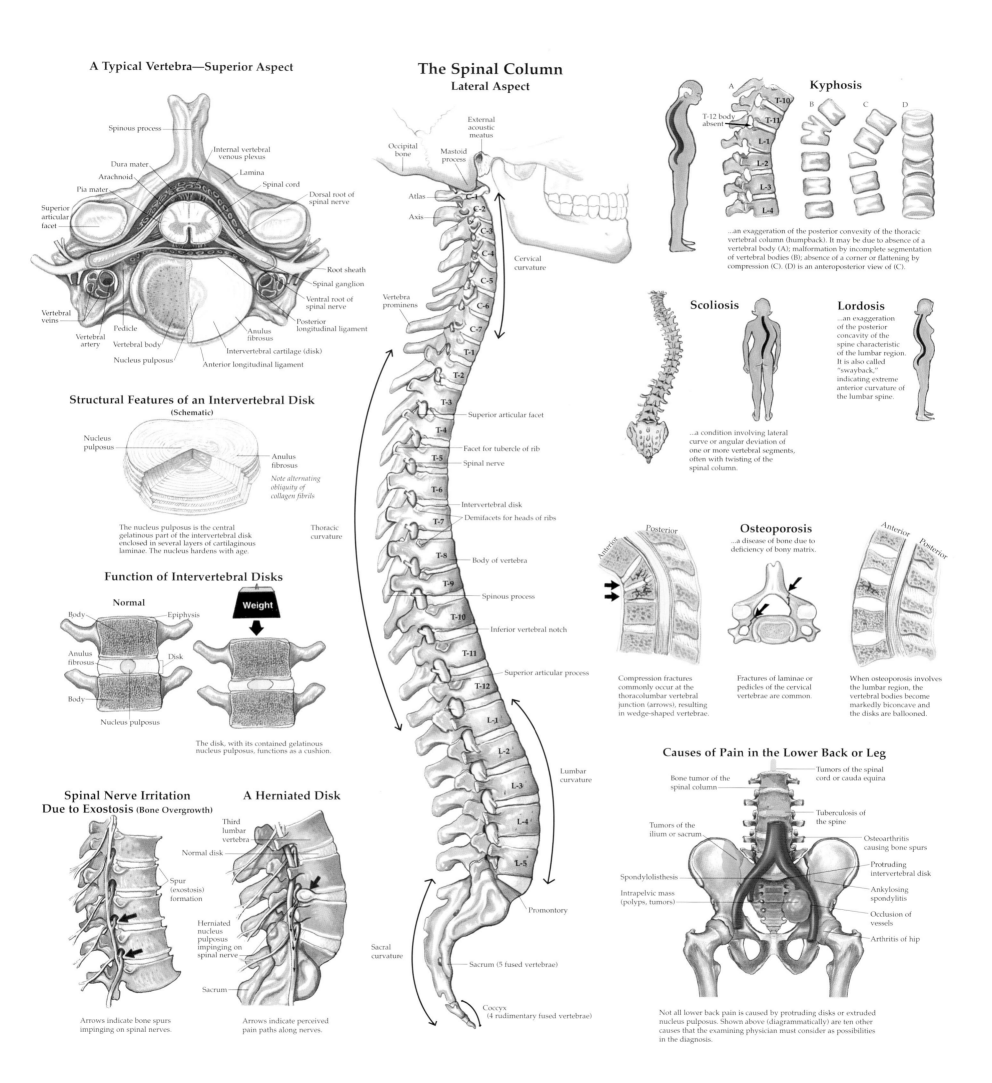

A Typical Vertebra—Superior Aspect

Spinous process
Internal vertebral venous plexus
Dura mater
Arachnoid
Lamina
Pia mater
Spinal cord
Superior articular facet
Dorsal root of spinal nerve
Root sheath
Spinal ganglion
Ventral root of spinal nerve
Vertebral veins
Posterior longitudinal ligament
Vertebral artery
Pedicle
Anulus fibrosus
Vertebral body
Intervertebral cartilage (disk)
Nucleus pulposus
Anterior longitudinal ligament

Structural Features of an Intervertebral Disk
(Schematic)

Nucleus pulposus
Anulus fibrosus
Note alternating obliquity of collagen fibrils

The nucleus pulposus is the central gelatinous part of the intervertebral disk enclosed in several layers of cartilaginous laminae. The nucleus hardens with age.

Function of Intervertebral Disks

Normal

Body
Epiphysis
Anulus fibrosus
Disk
Body
Nucleus pulposus

Weight

The disk, with its contained gelatinous nucleus pulposus, functions as a cushion.

Spinal Nerve Irritation Due to Exostosis (Bone Overgrowth)

Spur (exostosis) formation

Arrows indicate bone spurs impinging on spinal nerves.

A Herniated Disk

Third lumbar vertebra
Normal disk
Herniated nucleus pulposus impinging on spinal nerve
Sacrum

Arrows indicate perceived pain paths along nerves.

The Spinal Column
Lateral Aspect

External acoustic meatus
Occipital bone
Mastoid process
Atlas
Axis
Cervical curvature
Vertebra prominens
C-1
C-2
C-3
C-4
C-5
C-6
C-7
T-1
T-2
T-3
Superior articular facet
T-4
Facet for tubercle of rib
T-5
Spinal nerve
T-6
Intervertebral disk
T-7
Demifacets for heads of ribs
T-8
Body of vertebra
T-9
Spinous process
T-10
Inferior vertebral notch
T-11
T-12
Superior articular process
Thoracic curvature
L-1
L-2
L-3
L-4
Lumbar curvature
L-5
Promontory
Sacral curvature
Sacrum (5 fused vertebrae)
Coccyx (4 rudimentary fused vertebrae)

Kyphosis

...an exaggeration of the posterior convexity of the thoracic vertebral column (humpback). It may be due to absence of a vertebral body (A); malformation by incomplete segmentation of vertebral bodies (B); absence of a corner or flattening by compression (C). (D) is an anteroposterior view of (C).

T-10
T-11
T-12 body absent
L-1
L-2
L-3
L-4

Scoliosis

...a condition involving lateral curve or angular deviation of one or more vertebral segments, often with twisting of the spinal column.

Lordosis

...an exaggeration of the posterior concavity of the spine characteristic of the lumbar region. It is also called "swayback," indicating extreme anterior curvature of the lumbar spine.

Osteoporosis

...a disease of bone due to deficiency of bony matrix.

Posterior
Anterior

Compression fractures commonly occur at the thoracolumbar vertebral junction (arrows), resulting in wedge-shaped vertebrae.

Fractures of laminae or pedicles of the cervical vertebrae are common.

Anterior
Posterior

When osteoporosis involves the lumbar region, the vertebral bodies become markedly biconcave and the disks are ballooned.

Causes of Pain in the Lower Back or Leg

Bone tumor of the spinal column
Tumors of the ilium or sacrum
Spondylolisthesis
Intrapelvic mass (polyps, tumors)
Tumors of the spinal cord or cauda equina
Tuberculosis of the spine
Osteoarthritis causing bone spurs
Protruding intervertebral disk
Ankylosing spondylitis
Occlusion of vessels
Arthritis of hip

Not all lower back pain is caused by protruding disks or extruded nucleus pulposus. Shown above (diagrammatically) are ten other causes that the examining physician must consider as possibilities in the diagnosis.

9970

21

HYPERTENSION

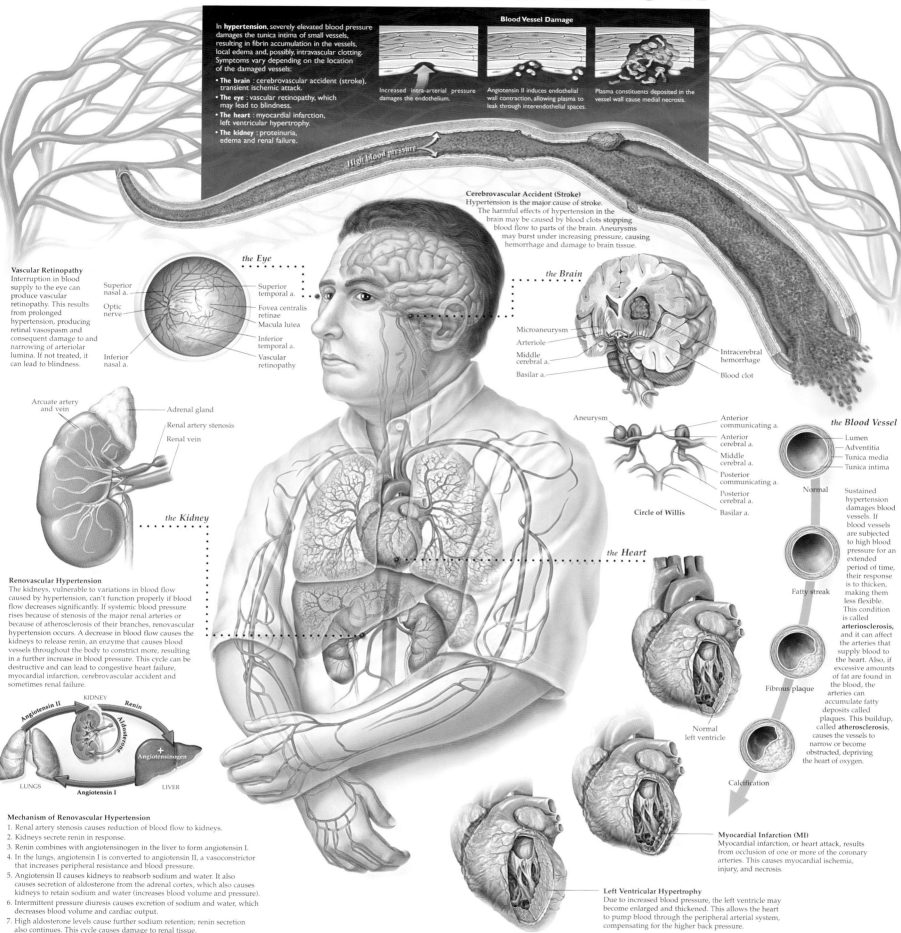

In **hypertension**, severely elevated blood pressure damages the tunica intima of small vessels, resulting in fibrin accumulation in the vessels, local edema and, possibly, intravascular clotting. Symptoms vary depending on the location of the damaged vessels:

- **The brain** : cerebrovascular accident (stroke), transient ischemic attack.
- **The eye** : vascular retinopathy, which may lead to blindness.
- **The heart** : myocardial infarction, left ventricular hypertrophy.
- **The kidney** : proteinuria, edema and renal failure.

Blood Vessel Damage

Increased intra-arterial pressure damages the endothelium.

Angiotensin II induces endothelial wall contraction, allowing plasma to leak through interendothelial spaces.

Plasma constituents deposited in the vessel wall cause medial necrosis.

High blood pressure

Cerebrovascular Accident (Stroke)
Hypertension is the major cause of stroke. The harmful effects of hypertension in the brain may be caused by blood clots stopping blood flow to parts of the brain. Aneurysms may burst under increasing pressure, causing hemorrhage and damage to brain tissue.

Vascular Retinopathy
Interruption in blood supply to the eye can produce vascular retinopathy. This results from prolonged hypertension, producing retinal vasospasm and consequent damage to and narrowing of arteriolar lumina. If not treated, it can lead to blindness.

the Eye

Superior nasal a.
Optic nerve
Inferior nasal a.
Superior temporal a.
Fovea centralis retinae
Macula lutea
Inferior temporal a.
Vascular retinopathy

the Brain

Microaneurysm
Arteriole
Middle cerebral a.
Basilar a.
Intracerebral hemorrhage
Blood clot

Aneurysm
Anterior communicating a.
Anterior cerebral a.
Middle cerebral a.
Posterior communicating a.
Posterior cerebral a.
Basilar a.

Circle of Willis

the Blood Vessel

Lumen
Adventitia
Tunica media
Tunica intima

Normal

Fatty streak

Fibrous plaque

Calcification

Arcuate artery and vein
Adrenal gland
Renal artery stenosis
Renal vein

the Kidney

Renovascular Hypertension
The kidneys, vulnerable to variations in blood flow caused by hypertension, can't function properly if blood flow decreases significantly. If systemic blood pressure rises because of stenosis of the major renal arteries or because of atherosclerosis of their branches, renovascular hypertension occurs. A decrease in blood flow causes the kidneys to release renin, an enzyme that causes blood vessels throughout the body to constrict more, resulting in a further increase in blood pressure. This cycle can be destructive and can lead to congestive heart failure, myocardial infarction, cerebrovascular accident and sometimes renal failure.

KIDNEY
Renin
Angiotensin II
Aldosterone
Angiotensinogen
LUNGS
LIVER
Angiotensin I

Mechanism of Renovascular Hypertension
1. Renal artery stenosis causes reduction of blood flow to kidneys.
2. Kidneys secrete renin in response.
3. Renin combines with angiotensinogen in the liver to form angiotensin I.
4. In the lungs, angiotensin I is converted to angiotensin II, a vasoconstrictor that increases peripheral resistance and blood pressure.
5. Angiotensin II causes kidneys to reabsorb sodium and water. It also causes secretion of aldosterone from the adrenal cortex, which also causes kidneys to retain sodium and water (increases blood volume and pressure).
6. Intermittent pressure diuresis causes excretion of sodium and water, which decreases blood volume and cardiac output.
7. High aldosterone levels cause further sodium retention; renin secretion also continues. This cycle causes damage to renal tissue.

the Heart

Normal left ventricle

Sustained hypertension damages blood vessels. If blood vessels are subjected to high blood pressure for an extended period of time, their response is to thicken, making them less flexible. This condition is called **arteriosclerosis**, and it can affect the arteries that supply blood to the heart. Also, if excessive amounts of fat are found in the blood, the arteries can accumulate fatty deposits called plaques. This buildup, called **atherosclerosis**, causes the vessels to narrow or become obstructed, depriving the heart of oxygen.

Myocardial Infarction (MI)
Myocardial infarction, or heart attack, results from occlusion of one or more of the coronary arteries. This causes myocardial ischemia, injury, and necrosis.

Left Ventricular Hypertrophy
Due to increased blood pressure, the left ventricle may become enlarged and thickened. This allows the heart to pump blood through the peripheral arterial system, compensating for the higher back pressure.

What Is Hypertension?
Hypertension or **high blood pressure** is a disorder marked by intermittent or consistent elevation of diastolic and/or systolic blood pressure. Generally, a sustained systolic pressure of 140 mm Hg or more, or a diastolic pressure of 90 mm Hg or more, qualifies as hypertension. The risk to the patient lies in the long-term damage that hypertension can cause to the brain, eyes, heart, blood vessels, and kidneys.

Types and Causes of Hypertension
Essential hypertension is the most common type of hypertension, yet its cause is unknown. Family medical history, race, stress, obesity, a diet high in sodium or saturated fat, use of tobacco and oral contraceptives, sedentary lifestyle and aging have been studied to determine their role in the development of hypertension.
Secondary hypertension may result from renal vascular disease, renal parenchymal disease, pheochromocytoma, Cushing's syndrome, diabetes mellitus, dysfunction of the thyroid or pituitary, pregnancy and some neurologic disorders.

Complications and Symptoms of Hypertension
Hypertension is the major cause of cerebrovascular accident, cardiac disease, and renal failure. In many cases symptoms are not present and the disorder is revealed during evaluation for another disorder or during routine blood pressure screening. When symptoms do occur, they reflect the effect of hypertension on the organ systems.

Some symptoms
- Headache in occipital region, which then subsides spontaneously.
- Dizziness and/or fatigue.
- Nosebleeds, bloody urine, weakness, blurred vision and chest pain are indicative of vascular involvement.
- Hypertensive retinopathy–hemorrhage, exudates, and papilledema (swelling of optic nerve as result of intracranial pressure).
- Stenosis or occlusion of carotid artery.
- Enlarged kidneys may point to polycystic disease, a cause of secondary hypertension.
- Systolic or diastolic blood pressure, or both, are elevated.

Diagnostic Tests
- **Urinalysis** may show protein, red blood cells, or white blood cells, suggesting renal disease, or Glucose in the urine suggests diabetes mellitus.
- **Excretory urography** may reveal renal atrophy.
- **Serum potassium** can indicate adrenal dysfunction.
- **Blood urea nitrogen** helps detect renal disease.

Treatment
Essential hypertension has no cure, although drugs and modifications in diet and lifestyle can usually control it. Treatment for secondary hypertension involves the correction of the underlying cause and controlling of hypertensive effects.

Drug treatments can include diuretics, beta-adrenergic blockers, calcium channel blockers, angiotensin converting enzyme inhibitors, and angiotensin receptor blockers (ARB's).

Healthy Lifestyle Changes
You may be able to decrease blood pressure by:
- Reducing body weight.
- Restricting dietary salt.
- Increasing fiber and decreasing fat in your diet.
- Not smoking.
- Avoiding excess alcohol.
- Exercising regularly.
- Practicing relaxation techniques.

It is very important to follow your physician's instructions and to take any medications as prescribed.

©2000 Anatomical Chart Company, a division of Springhouse Corporation.
Medical illustratons by Lik Kwong, M.F.A.

9767

KNEE INJURIES

Stability through a Range of Motion

The femur and the tibia are held tightly together by the tension of muscles crossing the joint, the joint capsule and four ligaments: anterior cruciate, posterior cruciate, fibular collateral and tibial collateral.

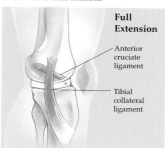

Full Extension

- Anterior cruciate ligament
- Tibial collateral ligament

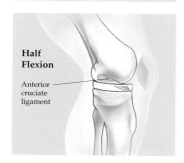

Half Flexion

- Anterior cruciate ligament

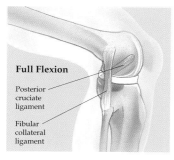

Full Flexion

- Posterior cruciate ligament
- Fibular collateral ligament

Normal Knee Anatomy
(Patella removed)

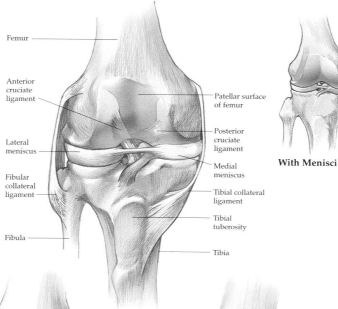

- Femur
- Anterior cruciate ligament
- Lateral meniscus
- Fibular collateral ligament
- Fibula
- Patellar surface of femur
- Posterior cruciate ligament
- Medial meniscus
- Tibial collateral ligament
- Tibial tuberosity
- Tibia

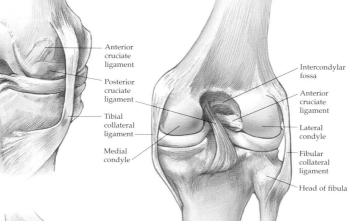

- Anterior cruciate ligament
- Posterior cruciate ligament
- Tibial collateral ligament
- Medial condyle
- Intercondylar fossa
- Anterior cruciate ligament
- Lateral condyle
- Fibular collateral ligament
- Head of fibula

Meniscus

The meniscus is a crescent-shaped piece of cartilage that lies between the femur and tibia. Each knee has two menisci, one medial and one lateral. Together, they cushion the joint by distributing downward forces outward and away from the central anchor points of the menisci.

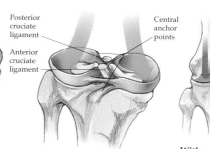

- Posterior cruciate ligament
- Anterior cruciate ligament
- Central anchor points

With Menisci   **Without Menisci**

Meniscus Tears

Rotation of the femur can pinch and tear the meniscus.

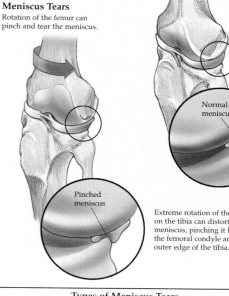

- Normal meniscus
- Pinched meniscus

Extreme rotation of the femur on the tibia can distort the meniscus, pinching it between the femoral condyle and the outer edge of the tibia.

Types of Meniscus Tears

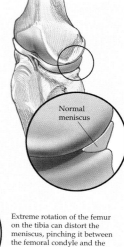

Oblique   Longitudinal   Transverse   Horizontal   Abrasion

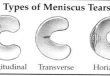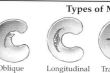

Traumatic Knee Injuries

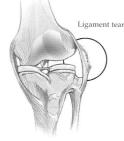

- Ligament tear

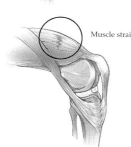

- Muscle strain

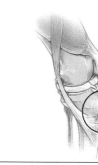

- Bone avulsion
- Ligament sprain

Symptoms of Damaged Menisci

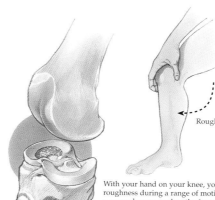

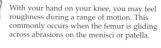

- Roughness

With your hand on your knee, you may feel roughness during a range of motion. This commonly occurs when the femur is gliding across abrasions on the menisci or patella.

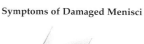

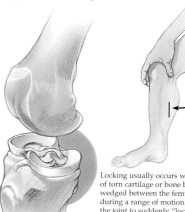

- Locking

Locking usually occurs when a piece of torn cartilage or bone becomes wedged between the femur and tibia during a range of motion. This causes the joint to suddenly "lock."

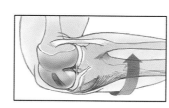

Sports Related Ligament Injuries

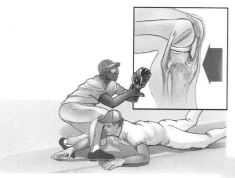

Sudden posterior movement of the tibia while the knee is flexed at 90° may damage the posterior cruciate ligament.

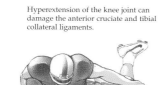

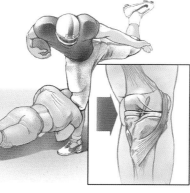

Hyperextension of the knee joint can damage the anterior cruciate and tibial collateral ligaments.

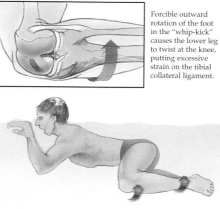

Forcible outward rotation of the foot in the "whip-kick" causes the lower leg to twist at the knee, putting excessive strain on the tibial collateral ligament.

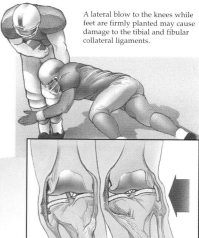

A lateral blow to the knees while feet are firmly planted may cause damage to the tibial and fibular collateral ligaments.

9872

©1993, 2000 Anatomical Chart Company, a division of Springhouse Corporation.
Medical illustrations by Birk Cox, in consultation with Alexander Kalenak, M.D.

UNDERSTANDING MENOPAUSE

What Is Menopause?

The word "menopause" is derived from the Greek words *men*, which means "monthly," and *pausis*, which means "ending." Literally, menopause refers to the complete ending of menstrual cycles, including ovulation, menstrual periods, and the possibility of pregnancy. In popular usage, "menopause" usually refers to the period of time in a woman's life from the first sign of menstrual irregularity to the time her body has completely adjusted to the changes. It is as natural an event as the onset of menstruation during puberty. It occurs any time between the ages of 40 and 60, usually beginning around age 50.

What Is Estrogen?

Estrogen is a hormone, a chemical substance secreted into body fluids that exerts an effect on specific cells of the body. The principal source of estrogen during a woman's reproductive years is her ovaries.

The ovaries contain 500,000 follicles, or egg cells, at birth. After the onset of puberty, about 20 follicles begin to develop each month and secrete estrogen. This estrogen stimulates further enlargement of these follicles until one outgrows the others and ovulates, releasing an egg into the fallopian tube. The empty follicle, called a corpus luteum, continues to secrete high amounts of estrogen, causing the uterine lining to become thick and vascular. If fertilization of the egg does not occur, this lining is shed during menstruation.

Effects of Estrogen

During puberty, the ovaries begin to secrete high amounts of estrogen. Estrogen prepares a woman's body for fertilization of an egg and nourishment of the resulting embryo. It also creates feminine characteristics of the body.

Female Physique
- Fat deposition in breasts and other areas
- Growth of stromal tissues and ductile system in breasts
- Growth of female pubic hair

Female Reproductive System
- Size of reproductive organs increases after puberty
- Vaginal mucosa becomes more resistant to trauma and infection
- Growth of hairlike cilia in fallopian tubes, which always beat toward the uterus

Skeletal System
- Calcium retention increases, promoting bone growth
- Pelvic opening enlarges from a narrow funnel to a broad oval

Other Effects
- Metabolism and total body protein increase
- Skin becomes thicker and more vascular

Birth Control During Menopause

Age at last period	Use birth control
50 or younger	2 years after last period
Older than 50	1 year after last period

Uterus

Proper ovarian ligament

Uterine (fallopian) tube

Uterine (fallopian) tube

Fimbria

Egg

Corpus luteum

Developing follicles

During Reproductive Years
Many active follicles secrete estrogen.

Follicles

Ovary of an infant

Ovary of a post-menopausal woman

Degenerating follicles

Developing follicles

Fewer follicles

Ovary

Levels of Estrogen
- First ovulation
- First period
- Last period

Birth 10 20 30 40 50 60 70 80
Age, in years

Early Menopause
Estrogen levels too low to complete cycle consistently.

At the onset of menopause, many of the follicles in the ovaries have either been "used up" or have degenerated over time. Estrogen production goes down as the number of follicles decreases. When estrogen levels fall below a critical value, ovulation cannot occur consistently, and menstrual periods become irregular. Eventually, all follicles degenerate and reproductive cycles stop altogether.

Body Changes

Hair Growth
- Thinning of scalp hair
- Darkening or thickening of other body hair, such as facial hair

Skin
- Loss of firmness, tension, and fluid
- Decrease in melanocytes, which give skin pigment
- Increased sensitivity to sun exposure

Bone
- Becomes progressively more porous and brittle
- Increased risk of osteoporosis
- More subject to fractures, especially the shoulder, upper arm, and hip

Breasts
- Glandular tissue replaced with fat
- Flattening of form

Suspensory ligaments

Fat

Gland lobules

Reproductive System
- Few remaining follicles (egg cells) in ovaries
- Reproductive organs decrease in size
- Vaginal mucosa becomes thinner, less lubricated
- Vaginal pH changes, increasing susceptibility to infection
- Endometriosis disappears

Ureter

Uterus

Ovary

Bladder

Vagina

Urethra

Urinary System
- Thinning of tissues in bladder and urethra
- Increased risk of urinary tract infections

Symptoms

During menopause, estrogen production does not stop completely. Post-menopausal estrogen levels are about 75% lower than during reproductive years. Symptoms experienced during menopause are the body's response to this decrease.

Irregular Menstruation
Irregularity of menstrual periods is the earliest, most common symptom of menopause. Normal changes include longer or shorter periods, excessive or minimal bleeding, spotting between periods, or skipping periods. Once you experience a six-month lapse in menstrual periods, there is a 90% chance menstruation will not resume.

Painful Intercourse
Lower estrogen levels can cause thinning of vaginal tissues and a decrease in lubricating fluid, leading to uncomfortable or painful intercourse. Using a lubricant during intercourse may alleviate this discomfort.

Hot Flashes, Night Sweats, and Insomnia
Hot flashes, a warm feeling in the face and neck that sometimes spreads to the back or chest, may happen throughout the day and night, causing discomfort and interfering with restful sleep. Hot flashes are caused by low estrogen levels but are not completely understood. For an unknown reason, the brain gets a message that the body is too hot and triggers a reflex response that dilates blood vessels near the skin, causing it to sweat and give off heat. Although hot flashes are uncomfortable, they are not dangerous and are usually unnoticed by others.

No Symptoms
Some women experience no symptoms other than cessation of menstrual periods.

Vaginal Mucosa

Menopause

Reproductive Years

Cornified cells
Intermediate cells
Parabasal cells

Other Symptoms
- Muscle and joint pain
- Backaches
- Depression
- Nervousness
- Irritability
- Headaches
- Fatigue
- Dizziness
- Urinary incontinence
- Formication (prickling or itching sensations of the skin)
- Palpitations (periods of rapid heartbeat)

Although all of these occurrences are normal, it is important to see your doctor regularly to discuss your symptoms.

Heat escapes

Epidermis of skin

Sweat

Dilated blood vessel

25% NO SYMPTOMS
50% MINOR SYMPTOMS
25% MANY INCONVENIENT SYMPTOMS

Estrogen Replacement Therapy

Estrogen replacement therapy (ERT) can relieve hot flashes and stop thinning of the vaginal mucosa. At slightly higher doses, ERT can decrease the risk of osteoporosis and heart disease. It is also true, however, that some research has suggested a link between breast cancer and ERT. It is a woman's individual decision whether or not to receive treatment. Are the symptoms of menopause interfering with your quality of life? What is your family history of osteoporosis and heart disease? Would taking ERT create an overriding fear of cancer? These are good questions to discuss with your doctor.

The Change of Life

Menopause can be a natural, positive experience for a woman, representing a new stage of life and sexual freedom. At current life expectancy figures, one third of a woman's life is spent in post-menopausal years. It is important to be good to your body during this time. Be sure to engage in weight-bearing exercise, such as walking and jogging, several times a week to slow loss of bone mass. Include calcium-rich foods such as skim milk, broccoli, and spinach in your daily diet. In addition to improving physical health, frequent exercise and a balanced diet can contribute to a feeling of well-being.

©1995, 2000 Anatomical Chart Company, a division of Springhouse Corporation.
Medical illustrations by Claudia M. Grosz, C.M.I., in consultation with Marko Jachtorowycz, M.D.

9977

MIDDLE EAR CONDITIONS

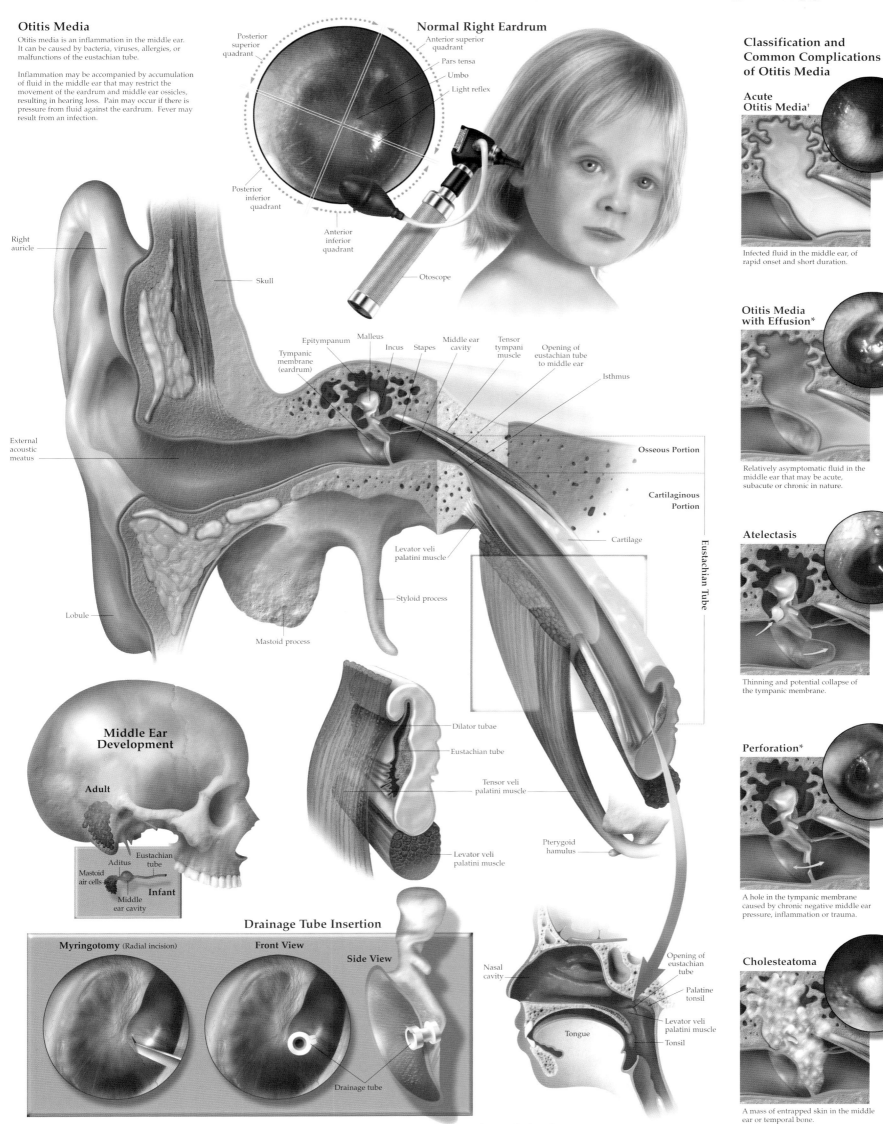

Otitis Media

Otitis media is an inflammation in the middle ear. It can be caused by bacteria, viruses, allergies, or malfunctions of the eustachian tube.

Inflammation may be accompanied by accumulation of fluid in the middle ear that may restrict the movement of the eardrum and middle ear ossicles, resulting in hearing loss. Pain may occur if there is pressure from fluid against the eardrum. Fever may result from an infection.

Normal Right Eardrum

- Posterior superior quadrant
- Anterior superior quadrant
- Pars tensa
- Umbo
- Light reflex
- Posterior inferior quadrant
- Anterior inferior quadrant
- Otoscope

- Right auricle
- Skull
- Epitympanum
- Malleus
- Incus
- Stapes
- Middle ear cavity
- Tensor tympani muscle
- Opening of eustachian tube to middle ear
- Tympanic membrane (eardrum)
- Isthmus
- Osseous Portion
- Cartilaginous Portion
- Cartilage
- External acoustic meatus
- Levator veli palatini muscle
- Eustachian Tube
- Styloid process
- Lobule
- Mastoid process

Middle Ear Development

- Adult
- Aditus
- Eustachian tube
- Mastoid air cells
- Middle ear cavity
- Infant

- Dilator tubae
- Eustachian tube
- Tensor veli palatini muscle
- Levator veli palatini muscle
- Pterygoid hamulus

Drainage Tube Insertion

- Myringotomy (Radial incision)
- Front View
- Side View
- Drainage tube

- Nasal cavity
- Opening of eustachian tube
- Palatine tonsil
- Levator veli palatini muscle
- Tongue
- Tonsil

Classification and Common Complications of Otitis Media

Acute Otitis Media[†]
Infected fluid in the middle ear, of rapid onset and short duration.

Otitis Media with Effusion*
Relatively asymptomatic fluid in the middle ear that may be acute, subacute or chronic in nature.

Atelectasis
Thinning and potential collapse of the tympanic membrane.

Perforation*
A hole in the tympanic membrane caused by chronic negative middle ear pressure, inflammation or trauma.

Cholesteatoma
A mass of entrapped skin in the middle ear or temporal bone.

UNDERSTANDING OSTEOPOROSIS

What is Osteoporosis?

Osteoporosis is a metabolic disease affecting the skeleton which causes a reduction in the amount of bone tissue. Bones are weakened as these tissues are resorbed or taken up by local cells. At the core, trabecular bone becomes less dense. On the perimeter, cortical bone loses thickness. Osteoporosis increases the bones susceptibility to fracture because of thinner bone tissue at the perimeter and more porous bone tissue in the core. Type I, Postmenopausal Osteoporosis, usually occurs in women following menopause. Type II, or Age-Related Osteoporosis, inflicts both women and men aged 70 or older.

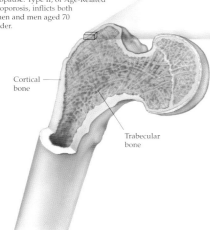

Normal bone

Osteoporotic bone

Cortical bone

Trabecular bone

Cortical bone

Trabecular bone

Bone Formation & Restoration

Bone is composed of 30% organic and 70% mineral substances. The organic portion is called **osteoid** and acts as the matrix or framework for the mineral part. Osteoid is produced by bone cells called **osteoblasts**. The mineral part consists of calcium and other valuable minerals and hardens upon the osteoid matrix. **Osteoclasts** are large bone cells which reshape mature bone by resorbing the mineral and organic components. Bone formation and resorption are normal, continuous processes.

In osteoporosis, there is an overall decrease in bone mass because resorption by osteoclasts exceeds bone formation. Osteoblasts continue to produce bone, but not to the same extent that it is being resorbed.

Osteoblasts

Osteoclasts

Osteoid matrix

Calcium minerals

Postmenopausal Osteoporosis

This type of osteoporosis usually occurs in women several years after menopause. At this time, women's ovaries produce less estrogen (a female sex hormone). In the absence of estrogen, bone resorption increases, dropping overall bone mass below the maintenance density level and risking fracture.

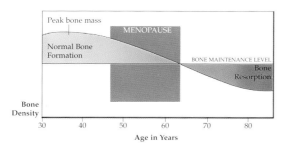

Peak bone mass

MENOPAUSE

Normal Bone Formation

BONE MAINTENANCE LEVEL

Bone Resorption

Bone Density

30   40   50   60   70   80

Age in Years

Age-Related Osteoporosis

Older age presents several additional concerns about osteoporosis. Adults over 70 have the added risk of low bone mass because bone density peaks at age 35 and decreases gradually. Secondly, the ability to absorb calcium from the intestine decreases, reducing calcium inside the body. Bone formation responds to physical stress, therefore, less activity decreases bone strength. Finally, older adults may be slightly Vitamin D deficient, also leading to decreased calcium absorption from the intestine. All of these factors predispose older people to osteoporosis and risk of bone fractures.

Effects of Osteoporosis

Osteoporosis may go unnoticed if it is asymptomatic. Symptoms of reduction in bone mass include:

• low back pain
• loss of height over time often accompanied by stooped posture
• minimal trauma fractures

As bone mass decreases, the risk of fracture grows.

Fractures of the proximal femur, or hip, may occur spontaneously or result from minor accidents. A femoral prosthesis can be used to repair a broken hip.

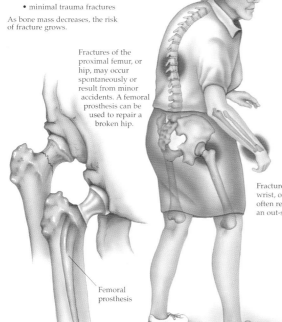

Femoral prosthesis

Controlling Your Mineral Balance

Calcium is normally absorbed by the blood from the digestive system and deposited into the bones. In osteoporosis, blood levels of calcium are slightly low due to dietary calcium deficiency, the inability of intestines to absorb calcium, or the lack of estrogen in the body as in postmenopause. To maintain calcium in the blood, resorption from the bones increases and causes osteoporosis.

In addition to enhanced bone resorption, low blood calcium increases the effects of two other factors: Parathyroid Hormone (PTH) and Vitamin D. Both stimulate calcium absorption from the intestine and increase resorption from bone. The result is an increased sacrifice of calcium in the bones to maintain normal levels of calcium in the blood.

Parathyroid glands are found behind the thyroid and produce PTH.

Parathyroid glands

Kidney

Normal absorption of calcium by intestines

Calcium

Ineffective absorption of calcium by intestines

Vitamin D is supplied by the diet and produced in the skin as a reaction to sunlight. It is processed into a very potent form in the liver and kidney.

Increased calcium resorption from bone

Ca^{++}

Calcium stored in bone

Ca^{++}

Osteoporotic bone

Normal bone

Compression fractures

in the lower spine result from a decrease in the trabecular bone of the vertebral bodies. They can be caused by little or no trauma. Deformities of the spine may occur due to a collapse of these injured vertebrae.

Fractures of the distal wrist, or Colles' fractures, often result from a fall on an out-stretched hand.

Dorsal kyphosis, or Dowager's Hump, often results from fractures to the front of the vertebral body. These wedge-shaped injuries are commonly associated with Age-Related Osteoporosis.

Compression fractures

Vertebral body

Vertebral disk

Keeping Bones Fit

Proper nutrition and a healthy lifestyle are important for the development and maintenance of bones. A physician can determine whether hormone replacement therapy is appropriate for each individual. Physical activity as a youth will build strong bones to last until old age. Eating a recommended daily calcium requirement and exercising will help maintain skeletal integrity and prevent potential bone fractures in the future.

9881

UNDERSTANDING PARKINSON'S DISEASE

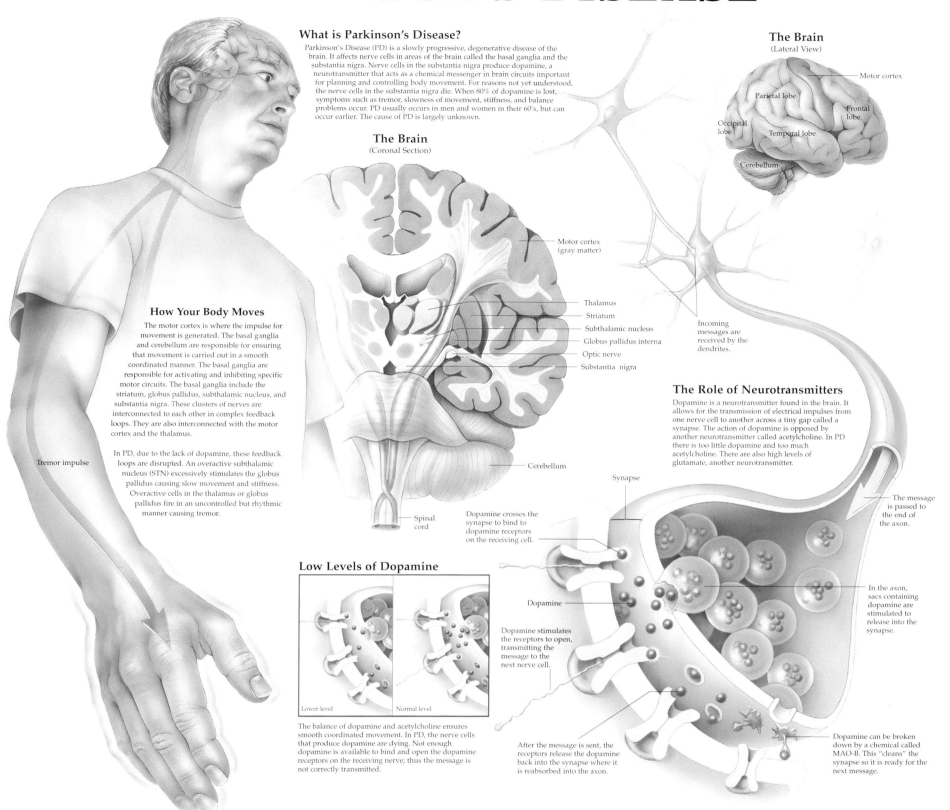

What is Parkinson's Disease?

Parkinson's Disease (PD) is a slowly progressive, degenerative disease of the brain. It affects nerve cells in areas of the brain called the basal ganglia and the substantia nigra. Nerve cells in the substantia nigra produce dopamine, a neurotransmitter that acts as a chemical messenger in brain circuits important for planning and controlling body movement. For reasons not yet understood, the nerve cells in the substantia nigra die. When 80% of dopamine is lost, symptoms such as tremor, slowness of movement, stiffness, and balance problems occur. PD usually occurs in men and women in their 60's, but can occur earlier. The cause of PD is largely unknown.

The Brain
(Lateral View)

Motor cortex
Parietal lobe
Occipital lobe
Temporal lobe
Frontal lobe
Cerebellum

The Brain
(Coronal Section)

Motor cortex (gray matter)
Thalamus
Striatum
Subthalamic nucleus
Globus pallidus interna
Optic nerve
Substantia nigra
Cerebellum
Spinal cord

Incoming messages are received by the dendrites.

How Your Body Moves

The motor cortex is where the impulse for movement is generated. The basal ganglia and cerebellum are responsible for ensuring that movement is carried out in a smooth coordinated manner. The basal ganglia are responsible for activating and inhibiting specific motor circuits. The basal ganglia include the striatum, globus pallidus, subthalamic nucleus, and substantia nigra. These clusters of nerves are interconnected to each other in complex feedback loops. They are also interconnected with the motor cortex and the thalamus.

In PD, due to the lack of dopamine, these feedback loops are disrupted. An overactive subthalamic nucleus (STN) excessively stimulates the globus pallidus causing slow movement and stiffness. Overactive cells in the thalamus or globus pallidus fire in an uncontrolled but rhythmic manner causing tremor.

Tremor impulse

The Role of Neurotransmitters

Dopamine is a neurotransmitter found in the brain. It allows for the transmission of electrical impulses from one nerve cell to another across a tiny gap called a synapse. The action of dopamine is opposed by another neurotransmitter called acetylcholine. In PD there is too little dopamine and too much acetylcholine. There are also high levels of glutamate, another neurotransmitter.

Synapse

The message is passed to the end of the axon.

Dopamine crosses the synapse to bind to dopamine receptors on the receiving cell.

Dopamine

In the axon, sacs containing dopamine are stimulated to release into the synapse.

Dopamine stimulates the receptors to open, transmitting the message to the next nerve cell.

Low Levels of Dopamine

Lower level   Normal level

The balance of dopamine and acetylcholine ensures smooth coordinated movement. In PD, the nerve cells that produce dopamine are dying. Not enough dopamine is available to bind and open the dopamine receptors on the receiving nerve; thus the message is not correctly transmitted.

After the message is sent, the receptors release the dopamine back into the synapse where it is reabsorbed into the axon.

Dopamine can be broken down by a chemical called MAO-B. This "cleans" the synapse so it is ready for the next message.

Medical Management

This is the first line of defense for PD patients. There are many options that may be used alone or in combination with each other to control symptoms.

1. Replace the missing dopamine in the brain. Levadopa enters the brain and is converted to dopamine. Carbidopa is used in combination to prevent breakdown of levadopa outside the brain which can cause nausea or irregularities of heart rhythm.

2. Optimize the delivery of levadopa to the brain by blocking COMT in the digestive system, allowing a steady supply of levadopa to reach the blood.

3. Block the breakdown of dopamine by MAO-B in the brain.

4. Introduce agents that mimic dopamine by binding to the dopamine receptors.

5. Reduce the activity of acetylcholine to bring the dopamine/acetylcholine activity in balance.

6. Block the excessive action of glutamate.

After a time on medication, patients may notice that each dose wears off before the next dose can be taken (wearing-off effect) or erratic fluctuations in dose effect (on-off effect). Another side effect patients may notice with time is dyskinesia, which are involuntary jerking or swaying movements of the body that typically occur at peak doses.

Surgical Management

When medical management fails due to fluctuations in the response, lack of effectiveness, or development of side effects such as dyskinesias, surgical options may be considered. These include destroying overactive areas of the brain or controlling them with electrical stimulation.

These procedures are done with a stereotactic frame attached to the skull. CT or MRI imaging is used to determine the exact location of the desired brain structure. Next, a small hole is made in the skull through which a probe is inserted into the brain structure.

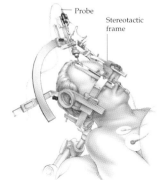

Probe
Stereotactic frame

Pallidotomy
The internal part of the globus pallidus interna (GPi) is destroyed by passing a high-frequency energy current which heats it to a desired temperature. This procedure is useful in controlling dyskinesias.

Thalamotomy
The same energy current is used to destroy a small area in the thalamus. This procedure is useful in controlling tremor.

Deep-Brain Stimulation (DBS)
An electrode is implanted in the desired area of the brain (globus pallidus, thalamus, or subthalamus), and then connected to a pacemaker implanted under the skin below the collar bone. The pacemaker sends electrical signals to regulate activity. Thalamic stimulation controls tremor; GPi or STN stimulation controls slowness of movement.

Symptoms

Symptoms may vary from person to person as does the rate of progression. The most common symptoms are listed below.

- Bradykinesia: Slowness of movement, impaired dexterity, decreased blinking, drooling, lack of facial expression.
- Tremor: Involuntary shaking, more prominent in resting position and decreases with purposeful movement.
- Rigidity: stiffness caused by increase in muscle tone.
- Postural Instability: sense of imbalance, tendency to fall.

Other symptoms that may or may not occur:
- Freezing
- Shuffling gait
- Stooped posture
- Small handwriting
- Insomnia
- Depression

Many people with Parkinson's enjoy an active lifestyle and a normal life expectancy. As yet there is no cure or definitive way to slow disease progression. However it is an area of ongoing research with new treatments constantly being developed.

Resources & Support

Contact the American Parkinsons Disease Association at 800-223-2732 or the National Parkinson Foundation at 800-327-4545 or the Parkinson's Disease Foundation at 800-457-6676 for local support groups and informational booklets.

9978

©2000 Anatomical Chart Company, a division of Springhouse Corporation. Written and illustrated by Tonya Hines, CMI and Tony Baker in consultation with Arif Dalvi, MD, The Neuroscience Institute Tristate Parkinson's Center, Cincinnati, Ohio.

THE RESPIRATORY SYSTEM & ASTHMA

Ventilation

Breathing or ventilation is the movement of air into and out of the respiratory system. During inspiration, the diaphragm and external intercostal muscles contract, causing the rib cage to expand and the volume of the thoracic cavity to increase. Air then rushes in to equalize the pressure. During expiration, the lungs passively recoil as the diaphragm and intercostal muscles relax, pushing air out of the lungs.

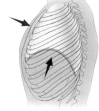

Inspiration
- Diaphragm contracts (moves down)
- Rib cage expands
- Lung volume increases

Expiration
- Diaphragm relaxes (moves up)
- Rib cage retracts
- Lung volume decreases

Gas Exchange

The respiratory unit consists of the respiratory bronchiole, alveolar duct, alveolar sac, and alveoli. Gas exchange occurs very rapidly in the millions of tiny, thin-membraned alveoli within the respiratory units. Inside these air sacs, oxygen from inhaled air diffuses into the blood as carbon dioxide diffuses from the blood into the air and is exhaled. Blood then circulates throughout the body, delivering oxygen and picking up carbon dioxide, then returning to the lungs to be oxygenated again.

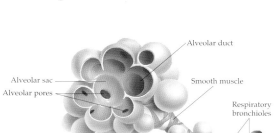

Alveolar duct
Alveolar sac
Alveolar pores
Smooth muscle
Respiratory bronchioles
Pulmonary artery
Alveoli
Pulmonary vein
Capillary beds cover all alveoli

Conducting System

The conducting system comprises all of the pathways through which air travels to reach the lungs. These pathways include the nasal cavity, pharynx, larynx, trachea, and bronchi. Within the conducting system, air is warmed, filtered, moistened, and delivered to and from the gas exchange area of the lungs.

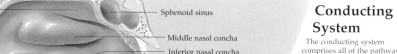
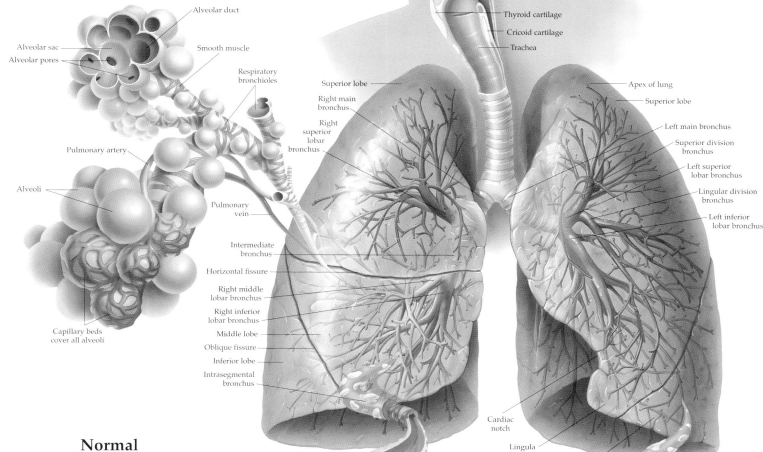

Frontal sinus
Superior nasal concha
Sphenoid sinus
Nasal cavity
Middle nasal concha
Inferior nasal concha
Opening of eustachian tube
Vestibule of nose
Nasopharynx
Soft palate
Oral cavity
Oropharynx
Epiglottis
Hyoid bone
Esophagus
Thyroid cartilage
Cricoid cartilage
Trachea
Superior lobe
Right main bronchus
Right superior lobar bronchus
Apex of lung
Superior lobe
Left main bronchus
Superior division bronchus
Left superior lobar bronchus
Lingular division bronchus
Left inferior lobar bronchus
Intermediate bronchus
Horizontal fissure
Right middle lobar bronchus
Right inferior lobar bronchus
Middle lobe
Oblique fissure
Inferior lobe
Intrasegmental bronchus
Cardiac notch
Lingula
Inferior lobe
Intrasegmental Bronchus
Cartilage

Common Asthma Triggers

Allergens

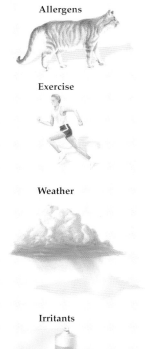

Exercise

Weather

Pollution

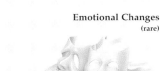

Irritants

Illness

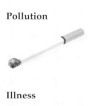

Emotional Changes (rare)

Normal Bronchiole

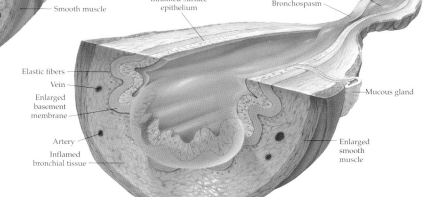

Elastic fibers
Vein
Surface epithelium
Basement membrane
Artery
Mucous gland
Smooth muscle

Asthmatic Bronchiole

Mucus plug
Bronchospasm
Inflamed surface epithelium
Elastic fibers
Vein
Enlarged basement membrane
Artery
Inflamed bronchial tissue
Mucous gland
Enlarged smooth muscle

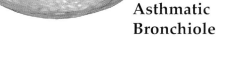

9768

UNDERSTANDING SKIN CANCER

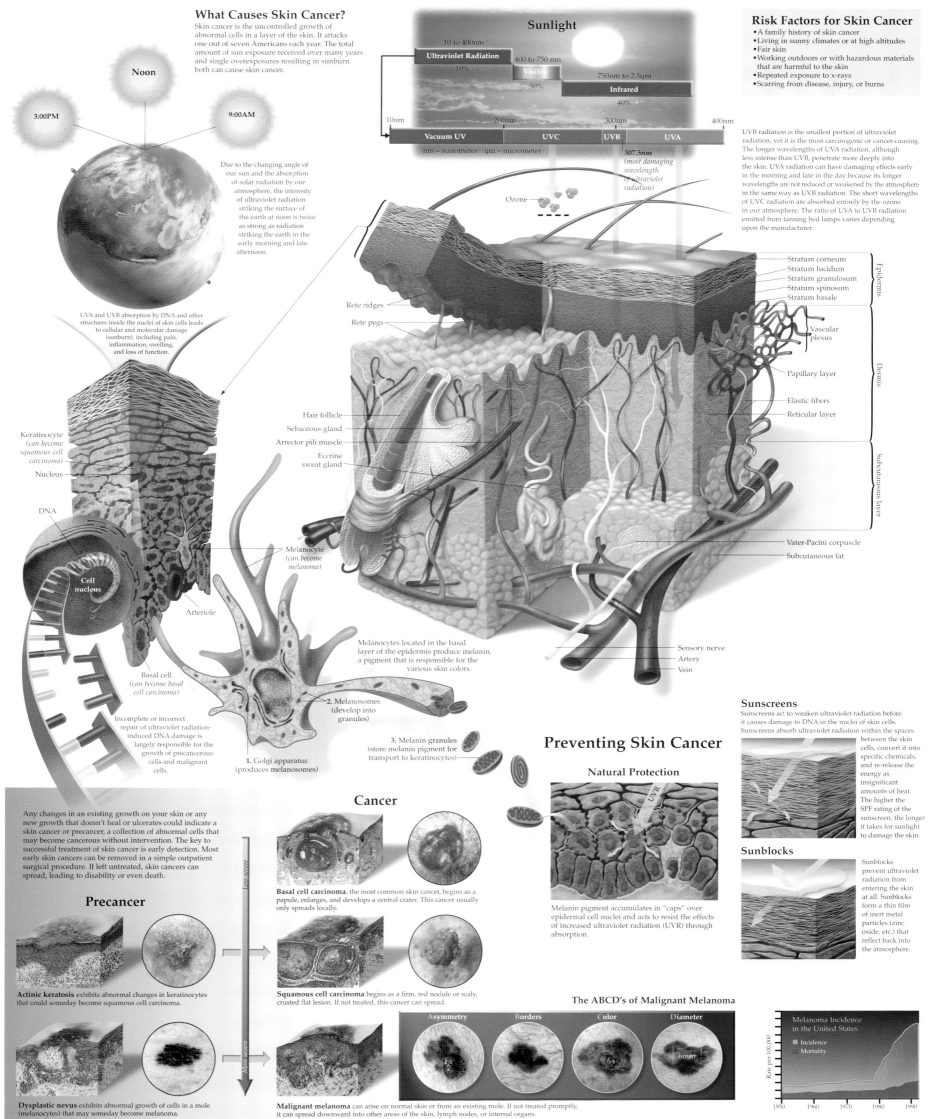

What Causes Skin Cancer?

Skin cancer is the uncontrolled growth of abnormal cells in a layer of the skin. It attacks one out of seven Americans each year. The total amount of sun exposure received over many years and single overexposures resulting in sunburn both can cause skin cancer.

Noon

3:00PM

9:00AM

Due to the changing angle of our sun and the absorption of solar radiation by our atmosphere, the intensity of ultraviolet radiation striking the surface of the earth at noon is twice as strong as radiation striking the earth in the early morning and late afternoon.

UVA and UVB absorption by DNA and other structures inside the nuclei of skin cells leads to cellular and molecular damage (sunburn), including pain, inflammation, swelling, and loss of function.

Keratinocyte (can become squamous cell carcinoma)

Nucleus

DNA

Cell nucleus

Arteriole

Basal cell (can become basal cell carcinoma)

Incomplete or incorrect repair of ultraviolet radiation-induced DNA damage is largely responsible for the growth of precancerous cells and malignant cells.

Sunlight

Ultraviolet Radiation 10%
10 to 400nm

Visible 50%
400 to 750 nm

Infrared 40%
750nm to 2.5μm

10nm — Vacuum UV — 200nm — UVC — UVB — 300nm — UVA — 400nm

nm = nanometer   μm = micrometer

307.5nm (most damaging wavelength of ultraviolet radiation)

Ozone

Rete ridges

Rete pegs

Hair follicle
Sebaceous gland
Arrector pili muscle
Eccrine sweat gland

Stratum corneum
Stratum lucidum
Stratum granulosum
Stratum spinosum
Stratum basale
} Epidermis

Vascular plexus

Papillary layer

Elastic fibers
Reticular layer
} Dermis

Vater-Pacini corpuscle
Subcutaneous fat
} Subcutaneous layer

Sensory nerve
Artery
Vein

Melanocyte (can become melanoma)

Melanocytes located in the basal layer of the epidermis produce melanin, a pigment that is responsible for the various skin colors.

2. Melanosomes (develop into granules)

3. Melanin granules (store melanin pigment for transport to keratinocytes)

1. Golgi apparatus (produces melanosomes)

Risk Factors for Skin Cancer

- A family history of skin cancer
- Living in sunny climates or at high altitudes
- Fair skin
- Working outdoors or with hazardous materials that are harmful to the skin
- Repeated exposure to x-rays
- Scarring from disease, injury, or burns

UVB radiation is the smallest portion of ultraviolet radiation, yet it is the most carcinogenic or cancer-causing. The longer wavelengths of UVA radiation, although less intense than UVB, penetrate more deeply into the skin. UVA radiation can have damaging effects early in the morning and late in the day because its longer wavelengths are not reduced or weakened by the atmosphere in the same way as UVB radiation. The short wavelengths of UVC radiation are absorbed entirely by the ozone in our atmosphere. The ratio of UVA to UVB radiation emitted from tanning bed lamps varies depending upon the manufacturer.

Preventing Skin Cancer

Natural Protection

Melanin pigment accumulates in "caps" over epidermal cell nuclei and acts to resist the effects of increased ultraviolet radiation (UVR) through absorption.

Sunscreens

Sunscreens act to weaken ultraviolet radiation before it causes damage to DNA in the nuclei of skin cells. Sunscreens absorb ultraviolet radiation within the spaces between the skin cells, convert it into specific chemicals, and re-release the energy as insignificant amounts of heat. The higher the SPF rating of the sunscreen, the longer it takes for sunlight to damage the skin.

Sunblocks

Sunblocks prevent ultraviolet radiation from entering the skin at all. Sunblocks form a thin film of inert metal particles (zinc oxide, etc.) that reflect back into the atmosphere.

Cancer

Any changes in an existing growth on your skin or any new growth that doesn't heal or ulcerates could indicate a skin cancer or precancer, a collection of abnormal cells that may become cancerous without intervention. The key to successful treatment of skin cancer is early detection. Most early skin cancers can be removed in a simple outpatient surgical procedure. If left untreated, skin cancers can spread, leading to disability or even death.

Basal cell carcinoma, the most common skin cancer, begins as a papule, enlarges, and develops a central crater. This cancer usually only spreads locally.

Squamous cell carcinoma begins as a firm, red nodule or scaly, crusted flat lesion. If not treated, this cancer can spread.

Precancer

Actinic keratosis exhibits abnormal changes in keratinocytes that could someday become squamous cell carcinoma.

Dysplastic nevus exhibits abnormal growth of cells in a mole (melanocytes) that may someday become melanoma.

Less severe / More severe

The ABCD's of Malignant Melanoma

Asymmetry | Borders | Color | Diameter

6mm

Malignant melanoma can arise on normal skin or from an existing mole. If not treated promptly, it can spread downward into other areas of the skin, lymph nodes, or internal organs.

Melanoma Incidence in the United States

Rate per 100,000

■ Incidence
□ Mortality

1950   1960   1970   1980   1990

DANGERS OF SMOKING

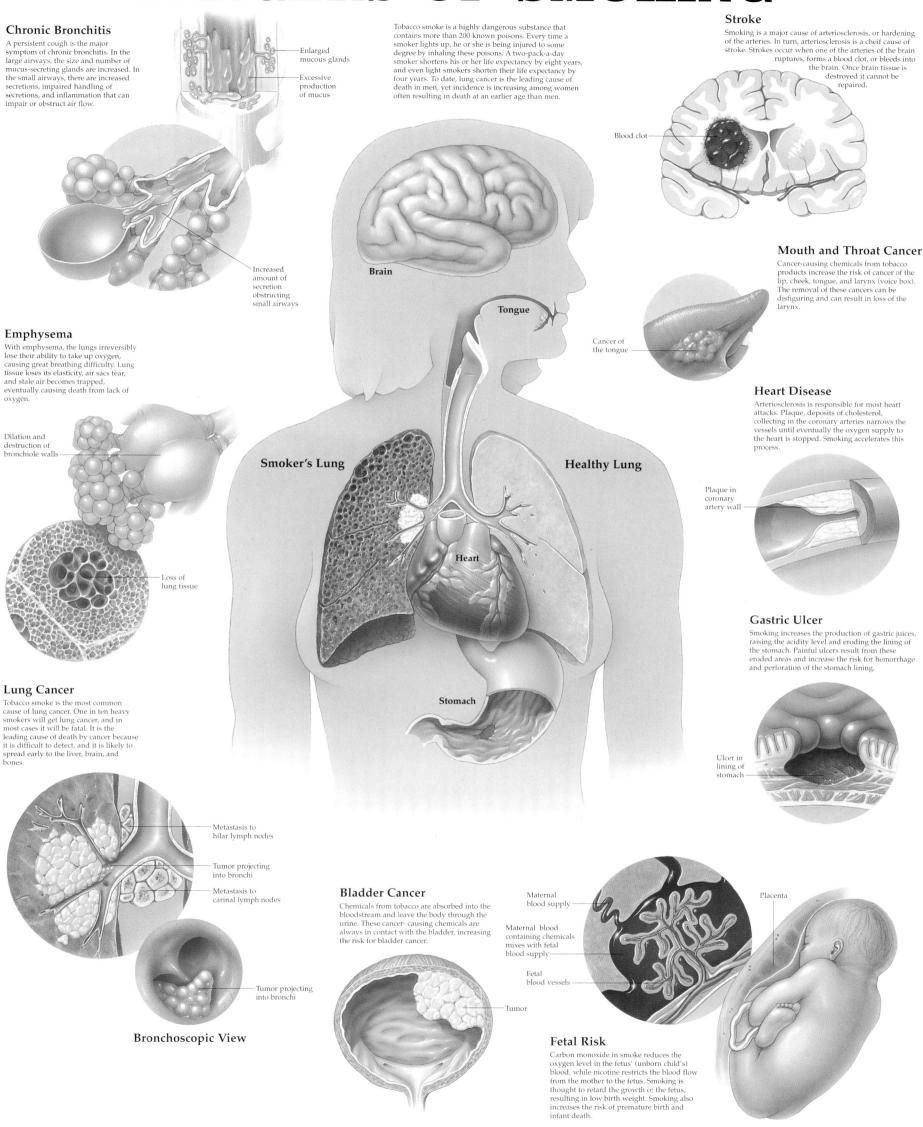

Chronic Bronchitis

A persistent cough is the major symptom of chronic bronchitis. In the large airways, the size and number of mucus-secreting glands are increased. In the small airways, there are increased secretions, impaired handling of secretions, and inflammation that can impair or obstruct air flow.

Enlarged mucous glands

Excessive production of mucus

Increased amount of secretion obstructing small airways

Emphysema

With emphysema, the lungs irreversibly lose their ability to take up oxygen, causing great breathing difficulty. Lung tissue loses its elasticity, air sacs tear, and stale air becomes trapped, eventually causing death from lack of oxygen.

Dilation and destruction of bronchiole walls

Loss of lung tissue

Lung Cancer

Tobacco smoke is the most common cause of lung cancer. One in ten heavy smokers will get lung cancer, and in most cases it will be fatal. It is the leading cause of death by cancer because it is difficult to detect, and it is likely to spread early to the liver, brain, and bones.

Metastasis to hilar lymph nodes

Tumor projecting into bronchi

Metastasis to carinal lymph nodes

Tumor projecting into bronchi

Bronchoscopic View

Tobacco smoke is a highly dangerous substance that contains more than 200 known poisons. Every time a smoker lights up, he or she is being injured to some degree by inhaling these poisons. A two-pack-a-day smoker shortens his or her life expectancy by eight years, and even light smokers shorten their life expectancy by four years. To date, lung cancer is the leading cause of death in men, yet incidence is increasing among women often resulting in death at an earlier age than men.

Brain

Tongue

Smoker's Lung

Healthy Lung

Heart

Stomach

Bladder Cancer

Chemicals from tobacco are absorbed into the bloodstream and leave the body through the urine. These cancer-causing chemicals are always in contact with the bladder, increasing the risk for bladder cancer.

Tumor

Stroke

Smoking is a major cause of arteriosclerosis, or hardening of the arteries. In turn, arteriosclerosis is a chief cause of stroke. Strokes occur when one of the arteries of the brain ruptures, forms a blood clot, or bleeds into the brain. Once brain tissue is destroyed it cannot be repaired.

Blood clot

Mouth and Throat Cancer

Cancer-causing chemicals from tobacco products increase the risk of cancer of the lip, cheek, tongue, and larynx (voice box). The removal of these cancers can be disfiguring and can result in loss of the larynx.

Cancer of the tongue

Heart Disease

Arteriosclerosis is responsible for most heart attacks. Plaque, deposits of cholesterol, collecting in the coronary arteries narrows the vessels until eventually the oxygen supply to the heart is stopped. Smoking accelerates this process.

Plaque in coronary artery wall

Gastric Ulcer

Smoking increases the production of gastric juices, raising the acidity level and eroding the lining of the stomach. Painful ulcers result from these eroded areas and increase the risk for hemorrhage and perforation of the stomach lining.

Ulcer in lining of stomach

Maternal blood supply

Maternal blood containing chemicals mixes with fetal blood supply

Fetal blood vessels

Placenta

Fetal Risk

Carbon monoxide in smoke reduces the oxygen level in the fetus' (unborn child's) blood, while nicotine restricts the blood flow from the mother to the fetus. Smoking is thought to retard the growth of the fetus, resulting in low birth weight. Smoking also increases the risk of premature birth and infant death.

9865

©1992, 2000 Anatomical Chart Company, a division of Springhouse Corporation.
Medical illustrations by Kimberly A. Martens, in consultation with
Russell M. Miller, M.D., F.A.A.F.P.

30

UNDERSTANDING STROKE

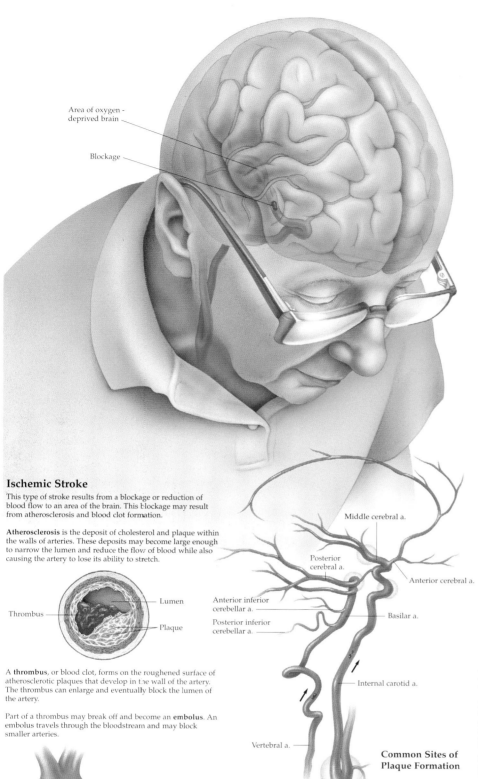

Area of oxygen - deprived brain

Blockage

What Is Stroke?

The term stroke refers to the sudden death of brain tissue caused by a lack of oxygen resulting from an interrupted blood supply. An **infarct** is the area of the brain that has "died" because of this lack of oxygen. There are two ways that brain tissue death can occur. **Ischemic stroke** is a blockage or reduction of blood flow in an artery that feeds that area of the brain. It is the most common cause of an infarct. **Hemorrhagic stroke** results from bleeding within and around the brain causing compression and tissue injury.

Events Leading to Stroke

Stroke victims often have small strokes or "warning sign," before a large permanent attack.

Transient Ischemic Attacks (TIAs) are brief attacks that last anywhere from a few minutes to 24 hours. The symptoms resolve completely and the person returns to normal. It is possible to have several TIAs before a large attack.
Reversible Ischemic Neurological Deficit (RIND) is an attack that lasts longer than 24 hours with recovery usually within three weeks. No tissue death occurs during a RIND, but the risk of a complete infarction is greatly increased after one.
Complete Infarction (CI) is an attack that leaves permanent tissue death and results in serious neurological deficits. Recovery is usually not total and takes longer than three weeks.

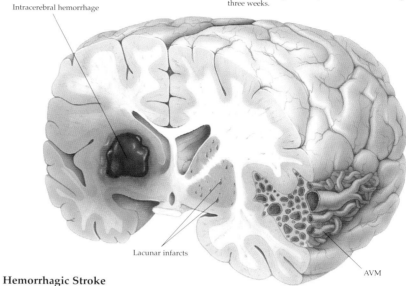

Intracerebral hemorrhage

Lacunar infarcts

AVM

Hemorrhagic Stroke

This type of stroke is caused by bleeding within and around the brain. Bleeding that fills the spaces between the brain and the skull is called a subarachnoid hemorrhage. It is caused by ruptured aneurysms, arteriovenous malformations, and head trauma. Bleeding within the brain tissue itself is known as intracerebral hemorrhage and is primarily caused by hypertension.

An **arteriovenous malformation** (AVM) is an abnormality of the brain's blood vessels in which arteries lead directly into veins without first going through a capillary bed. The pressure of the blood coming through the arteries is too high for the veins, causing them to dilate in order to transport the higher volume of blood. This dilation can cause them to rupture.

Ischemic Stroke

This type of stroke results from a blockage or reduction of blood flow to an area of the brain. This blockage may result from atherosclerosis and blood clot formation.

Atherosclerosis is the deposit of cholesterol and plaque within the walls of arteries. These deposits may become large enough to narrow the lumen and reduce the flow of blood while also causing the artery to lose its ability to stretch.

Thrombus — Lumen
— Plaque

A **thrombus**, or blood clot, forms on the roughened surface of atherosclerotic plaques that develop in the wall of the artery. The thrombus can enlarge and eventually block the lumen of the artery.

Part of a thrombus may break off and become an **embolus**. An embolus travels through the bloodstream and may block smaller arteries.

Bacterial endocarditis
Atrial fibrillation
Ball thrombus
Mitral valve stenosis
Embolus
Mural thrombi
Myocardial infarction

Emboli commonly come from the heart, where different diseases can cause thrombus formation.

Middle cerebral a.
Posterior cerebral a.
Anterior cerebral a.
Anterior inferior cerebellar a.
Posterior inferior cerebellar a.
Basilar a.
Internal carotid a.
Vertebral a.
Common carotid a.

Common Sites of Plaque Formation

Circle of Willis

Aneurysm

An **aneurysm** is a weakening of the arterial wall that causes it to stretch and balloon. It usually occurs where the artery branches.

Hypertension is an elevation of blood pressure that may cause tiny arterioles to burst in the brain. Blood released inside brain tissue puts pressure on adjacent arterioles, causing them to burst and lead to more bleeding. Hypertension may also cause lacunar infarcts. These are miniature infarcts similar to complete strokes, but on a much smaller scale. They occur within the nuclei and spinal tracts of the brain and resemble little lakes or pits.

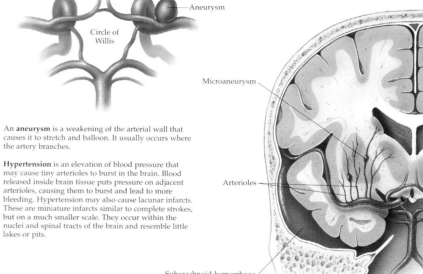

Microaneurysm
Arterioles
Subarachnoid hemorrhage

Motor strip
Sensory strip

Frontal lobe
Motor control of voluntary muscles
Personality
Concentration, organization
Problem-solving

Broca's center
Motor control of speech

Temporal lobe
Hearing
Memory of hearing and vision

Brain stem
Controls heart rate and rate of breathing

Parietal lobe
Sensory areas of touch, pain, temperature
Understanding speech, language
Express thoughts

Wernicke's center
Interpreting speech

Occipital lobe
Visual recognition
Focus the eye

Cerebellum
Balance
Coordinating muscle movement

Normal Functional Areas of Brain

The brain has two sides: a right hemisphere that controls the left side of the body and a left hemisphere that controls the right side of the body. Each hemisphere has four lobes and a cerebellum that control our daily functions. Depending on what part of the brain has been affected, stroke victims experience a variety of neurological deficits. Rehabilitation is crucial to the stroke patient's recovery. Physical therapists and speech therapists help patients "relearn" their lost functions and devise ways to cope with the loss of those they cannot regain.

What Increases Your Risk for Stroke?

Hypertension
Heart disease
Atherosclerosis
Previous TIAs
High cholesterol
High alcohol consumption
Obesity
Diabetes
Bruit noise in carotid artery
Cigarette smoking
Oral contraceptive use
Family history of stroke

Common Neurological Deficits After Stroke

Left-sided stroke	Right-sided stroke	Related Terms	
• Right-sided paralysis	• Left-sided paralysis	Paralysis	Loss of muscle function and sensation
• Speech/language deficits	• Spatial/perceptual deficits	Hemiparesis	Weakness of muscles on one side of body
• Slow, cautious behavior	• Quick, impulsive behavior	Hemianopsia	Loss of sight in half of visual field
• Hemianopsia of right visual field	• Hemianopsia of left visual field	Aphasia	Inability to understand or produce language
• Memory loss in language	• Memory loss in performance	Apraxia	Inability to control muscles; movement is uncoordinated and jerky
• Right-sided dysarthria	• Left-sided dysarthria	Dysarthria	Slurring of speech and "mouth droop" on one side of face due to muscle weakness
• Aphasia			
• Apraxia			

9868

DISORDERS OF THE TEETH AND JAW

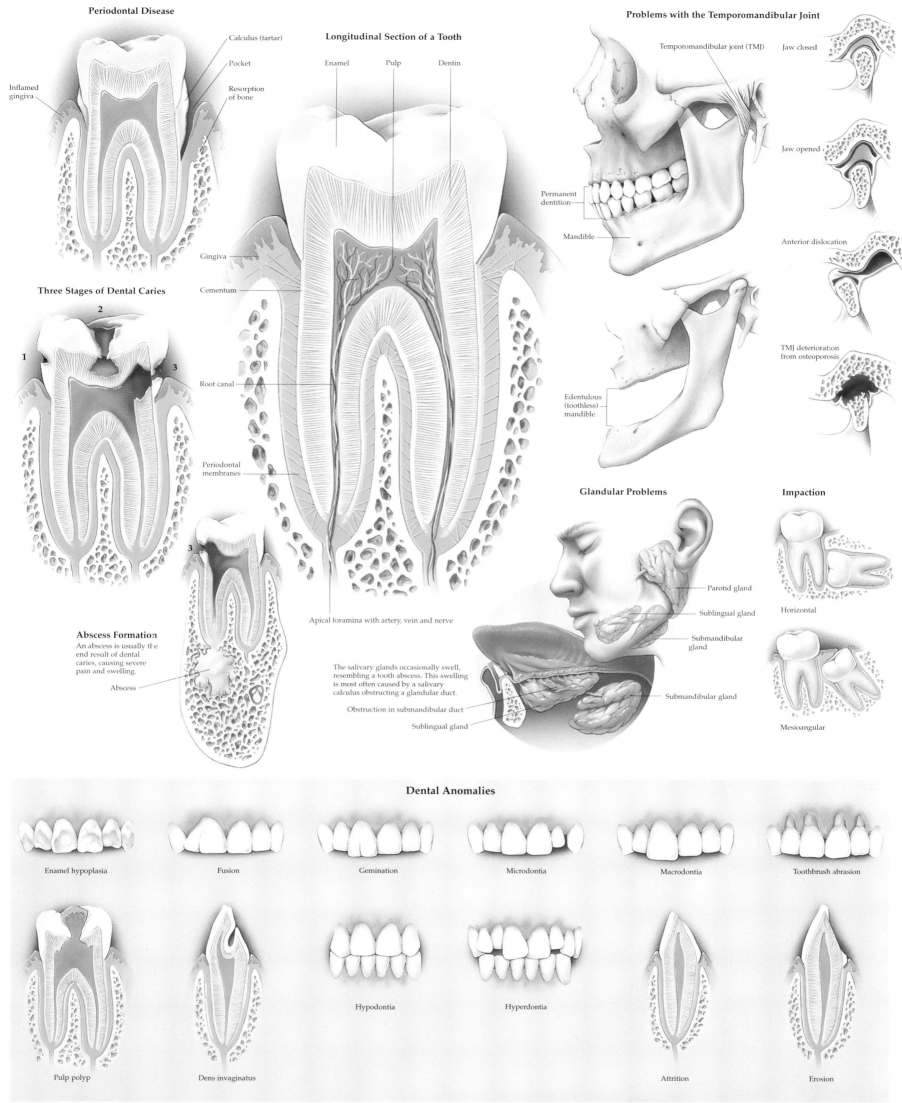

Periodontal Disease

Calculus (tartar)
Pocket
Resorption of bone
Inflamed gingiva

Longitudinal Section of a Tooth

Enamel
Pulp
Dentin
Gingiva
Cementum
Root canal
Periodontal membranes
Apical foramina with artery, vein and nerve

Problems with the Temporomandibular Joint

Temporomandibular joint (TMJ)
Jaw closed
Jaw opened
Anterior dislocation
TMJ deterioration from osteoporosis
Permanent dentition
Mandible
Edentulous (toothless) mandible

Three Stages of Dental Caries

1
2
3

Abscess Formation
An abscess is usually the end result of dental caries, causing severe pain and swelling.
Abscess

The salivary glands occasionally swell, resembling a tooth abscess. This swelling is most often caused by a salivary calculus obstructing a glandular duct.

Obstruction in submandibular duct
Sublingual gland

Glandular Problems

Parotid gland
Sublingual gland
Submandibular gland
Submandibular gland

Impaction

Horizontal
Mesioangular

Dental Anomalies

Enamel hypoplasia
Fusion
Gemination
Microdontia
Macrodontia
Toothbrush abrasion

Pulp polyp
Dens invaginatus
Hypodontia
Hyperdontia
Attrition
Erosion

9866

©1992, 2000 Anatomical Chart Company, a division of Springhouse Corporation.
Medical Illustrations by Craig L. Kiefer, in consultation with Dean P. Nicholas, D.D.S.

32

TEMPOROMANDIBULAR JOINT (TMJ)

Key: Muscles (m.)

A. Temporalis m.
B. Temporomandibular joint
C. Masseter m.
D. Stylohyoid m.
E. Digastric m. (posterior belly)
F. Longus capitis m.
G. Levator scapulae m.
H. Trapezius m.
I. Posterior scalene m.
J. Middle scalene m.
K. Sternocleidomastoid m.
L. Inferior pharyngeal constrictor m.
M. Thyrohyoid m.
N. Sternothyroid m.
O. Omohyoid m.
P. Sternohyoid m.
Q. Hyoglossus m.
R. Mylohyoid m.
S. Digastric m. (anterior belly)

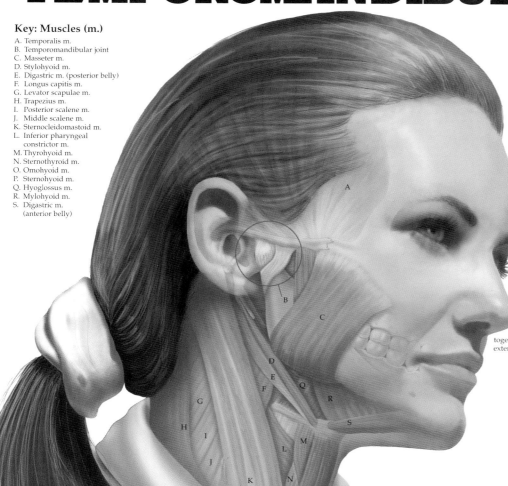

Normal Jaw (closed)

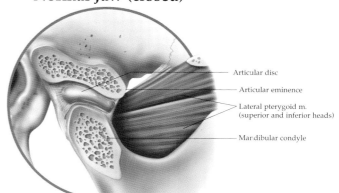

Articular disc
Articular eminence
Lateral pterygoid m. (superior and inferior heads)
Mandibular condyle

What is TMJ Syndrome?

TMJ syndrome is a term often used to describe a disorder of the temporomandibular joints (jaw joints) and/or the muscles that control the joints and balance the head on the spinal column. It is a collection of symptoms that occur when the jaw joints and/or surrounding muscles do not work together properly. The problem also can extend down the neck and back.

Normal Jaw (open)

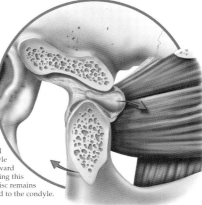

The purpose of the articular disc is to cushion the bones of the TMJ during opening and closing of the mouth. When the mouth opens, the mandibular condyle rotates on a horizontal axis. At the same time, the condyle and disc glide forward and downward on the articular eminence. During this entire motion the articular disc remains attached to the condyle.

Nerves of the Temporomandibular Region

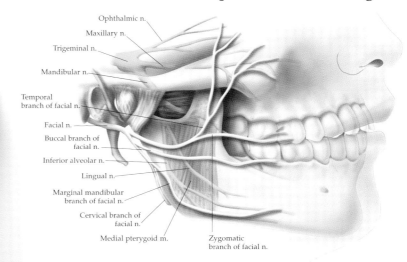

Ophthalmic n.
Maxillary n.
Trigeminal n.
Mandibular n.
Temporal branch of facial n.
Facial n.
Buccal branch of facial n.
Inferior alveolar n.
Lingual n.
Marginal mandibular branch of facial n.
Cervical branch of facial n.
Medial pterygoid m.
Zygomatic branch of facial n.

Common TMJ Syndrome Causes and Disorders

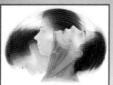

Whiplash

Whiplash causes the muscles of the neck to be jarred and pulled violently, often resulting in ligament tears, stretching of structures to their limits and discal tearing. All can lead to the development of TMJ symptoms.

Malocclusion

Malocclusion is the abnormal contact of opposing teeth with respect to the temporomandibular joint that interferes with the efficient movement of the jaw during mastication. It is one of the most frequent triggers of TMJ syndrome. Malocclusion, even on a minute scale can trigger the spasm of muscles, resulting in pain.

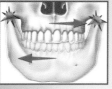

Bruxism/Clenching

Bruxism, the grinding of teeth, usually occurs during sleep. Clenching can occur throughout the day or night. Both can be directly related to TMJ, either as a trigger for muscle spasms or as a result of malocclusion. Constant grinding also causes pressure on the TMJ. Bruxing can put pressure on the articular disc, squeezing out synovial fluid and robbing it of lubrication.

Systemic Diseases

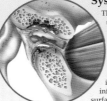

The TMJ, like any other joint, is susceptible to any of the systemic diseases. Immune disorders such as osteoarthritis, rheumatoid arthritis, psoriatic arthritis and systemic lupus erythematosus and electrolyte imbalances can produce inflammation and muscle cramping in the TMJ. In addition, viral infections can cause damage to the surfaces of the TMJ.

Loss of Teeth

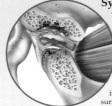

When a tooth is lost, the teeth around it tend to shift to fill the space. This change can alter the way the teeth gear in relation to the joint, causing symptoms to develop.

Disc Displacement

The jaw joint, in addition to being a ball and socket joint, glides forward and backward. When functioning correctly, the articular cartilage lies between the condyle head of the mandible and the roof of the joint. It normally follows the condylar head in its forward and backward movement. If the ligaments that hold the disc to the condylar head are injured, the disc can slip out of place and can no longer serve as a normal cushion between the lower and upper parts of the jaw. Typically, the disc is pulled forward. Mild displacements can cause a clicking or popping sound in the joint and sometimes can be painful. Permanent damage may result from the displacements.

Symptoms

Extracapsular- Outside the jaw joint.

- Headaches
- Tooth pain (caused by bruxism)
- Numbness or tingling of fingers
- Dizziness
- Neck, shoulder or back pain
- Pain behind eyes
- Earaches or ringing in ears

Intracapsular- Within the jaw joint.

- Crepitus (grinding sound)
- Clicking or popping
- Locking or limited range of motion
- Pain in and around jaw joints

Disorders Sometimes Mistaken for TMJ Syndrome

- Migraine headache
- Chemical allergies
- Temporal tendinitis
- Psychosomatic headache
- Ernest syndrome
- Sinusitis
- Brain tumors
- Trauma

Treatment

Phase 1- Attempts to break the cycle of muscle spasms, thereby relieving pain and producing a physiological relationship between the maxilla and mandible. Treatments can include:

- Use of an intra-oral orthotic or splint
- Anti-inflammatory medications
- Stress management
- Physical therapy
- Muscle relaxants
- Manipulative treatment

Phase 2- Attempts to break the cycle of pain through more permanent means of treatment. Treatments can include:

- Adjustment of dental occlusion
- Orthodontics
- Reconstruction of teeth
- Orthognathic surgery (surgical relocation of teeth or jaw)
- Replacement of missing teeth
- Surgery on TMJ itself (last resort)

9932

©2000 Anatomical Chart Company, a division of Springhouse Corporation.
Medical illustrations by Liana Bauman, MAMS in consultation with A. Richard Goldman, D.D.S.

UNDERSTANDING ULCERS

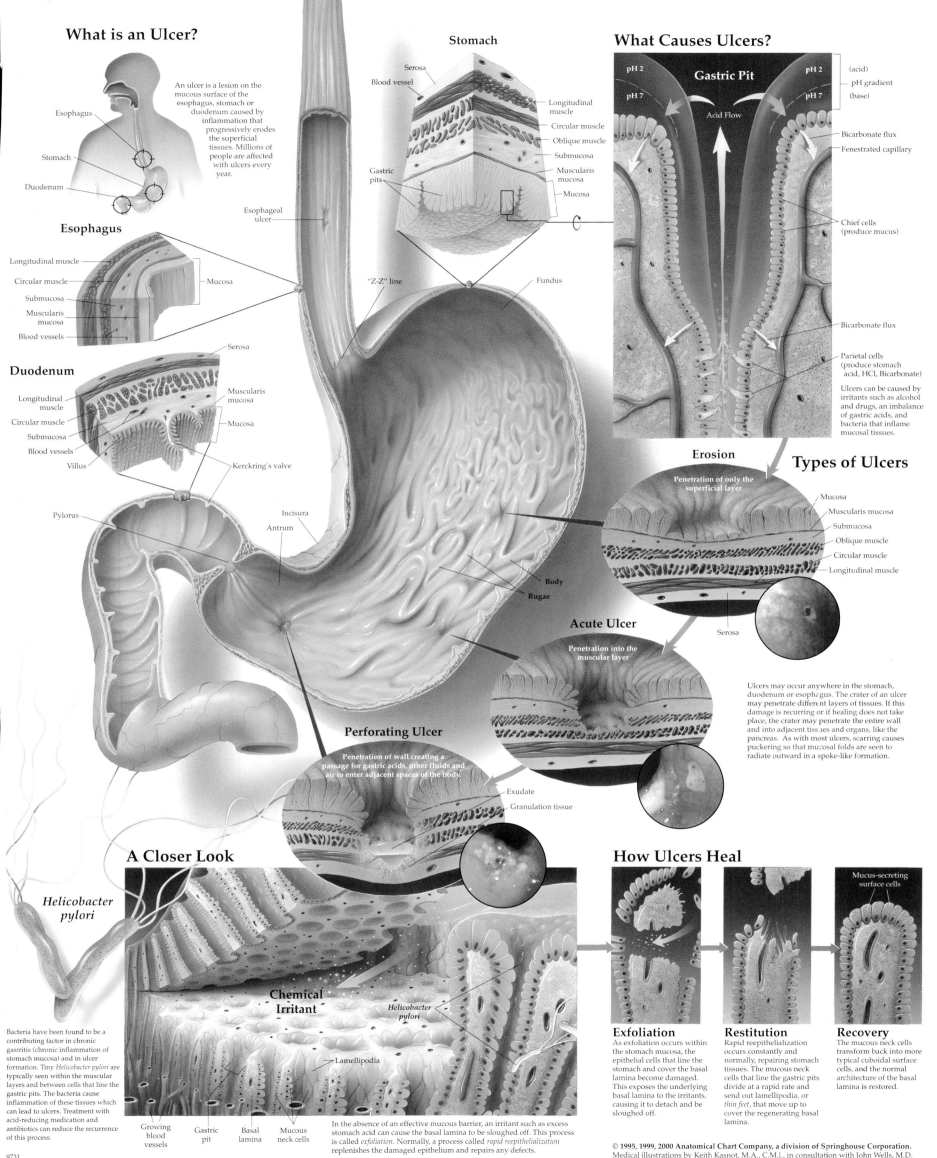

What is an Ulcer?

An ulcer is a lesion on the mucous surface of the esophagus, stomach or duodenum caused by inflammation that progressively erodes the superficial tissues. Millions of people are affected with ulcers every year.

Esophagus
Stomach
Duodenum

Esophagus

Longitudinal muscle
Circular muscle
Submucosa
Muscularis mucosa
Blood vessels
Mucosa

Duodenum

Longitudinal muscle
Circular muscle
Submucosa
Blood vessels
Villus
Serosa
Muscularis mucosa
Mucosa
Kerckring's valve

Pylorus
Incisura
Antrum

Stomach

Serosa
Blood vessel
Gastric pits
Longitudinal muscle
Circular muscle
Oblique muscle
Submucosa
Muscularis mucosa
Mucosa

Esophageal ulcer
"Z-Z" line
Fundus
Body
Rugae

What Causes Ulcers?

Gastric Pit
pH 2
pH 7
pH 2
pH 7
(acid)
pH gradient
(base)
Acid Flow

Bicarbonate flux
Fenestrated capillary
Chief cells (produce mucus)
Bicarbonate flux
Parietal cells (produce stomach acid, HCl, Bicarbonate)

Ulcers can be caused by irritants such as alcohol and drugs, an imbalance of gastric acids, and bacteria that inflame mucosal tissues.

Types of Ulcers

Erosion
Penetration of only the superficial layer

Mucosa
Muscularis mucosa
Submucosa
Oblique muscle
Circular muscle
Longitudinal muscle
Serosa

Acute Ulcer
Penetration into the muscular layer

Perforating Ulcer
Penetration of wall creating a passage for gastric acids, other fluids and air to enter adjacent spaces of the body.

Exudate
Granulation tissue

Ulcers may occur anywhere in the stomach, duodenum or esophagus. The crater of an ulcer may penetrate different layers of tissues. If this damage is recurring or if healing does not take place, the crater may penetrate the entire wall and into adjacent tissues and organs, like the pancreas. As with most ulcers, scarring causes puckering so that mucosal folds are seen to radiate outward in a spoke-like formation.

A Closer Look

Helicobacter pylori

Chemical Irritant

Helicobacter pylori
Lamellipodia

Bacteria have been found to be a contributing factor in chronic gastritis (chronic inflammation of stomach mucosa) and in ulcer formation. Tiny *Helicobacter pylori* are typically seen within the muscular layers and between cells that line the gastric pits. The bacteria cause inflammation of these tissues which can lead to ulcers. Treatment with acid-reducing medication and antibiotics can reduce the recurrence of this process.

Growing blood vessels
Gastric pit
Basal lamina
Mucous neck cells

In the absence of an effective mucous barrier, an irritant such as excess stomach acid can cause the basal lamina to be sloughed off. This process is called *exfoliation*. Normally, a process called *rapid reepithelialization* replenishes the damaged epithelium and repairs any defects.

How Ulcers Heal

Mucus-secreting surface cells

Exfoliation
As exfoliation occurs within the stomach mucosa, the epithelial cells that line the stomach and cover the basal lamina become damaged. This exposes the underlying basal lamina to the irritants, causing it to detach and be sloughed off.

Restitution
Rapid reepithelialization occurs constantly and normally, repairing stomach tissues. The mucous neck cells that line the gastric pits divide at a rapid rate and send out lamellipodia, or *thin feet*, that move up to cover the regenerating basal lamina.

Recovery
The mucous neck cells transform back into more typical cuboidal surface cells, and the normal architecture of the basal lamina is restored.

DISEASES OF THE URINARY TRACT

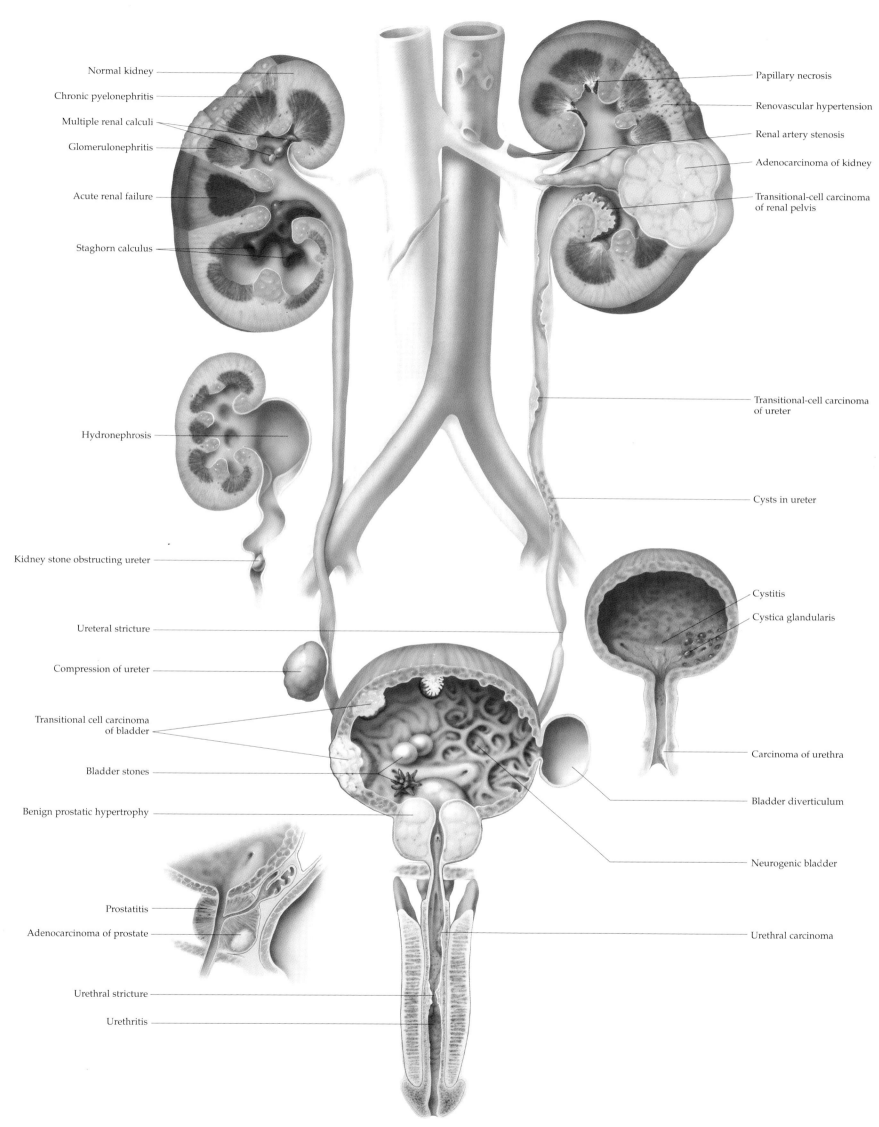

Normal kidney

Chronic pyelonephritis

Multiple renal calculi

Glomerulonephritis

Acute renal failure

Staghorn calculus

Hydronephrosis

Kidney stone obstructing ureter

Ureteral stricture

Compression of ureter

Transitional cell carcinoma of bladder

Bladder stones

Benign prostatic hypertrophy

Prostatitis

Adenocarcinoma of prostate

Urethral stricture

Urethritis

Papillary necrosis

Renovascular hypertension

Renal artery stenosis

Adenocarcinoma of kidney

Transitional-cell carcinoma of renal pelvis

Transitional-cell carcinoma of ureter

Cysts in ureter

Cystitis

Cystica glandularis

Carcinoma of urethra

Bladder diverticulum

Neurogenic bladder

Urethral carcinoma

WHIPLASH INJURIES OF THE HEAD AND NECK

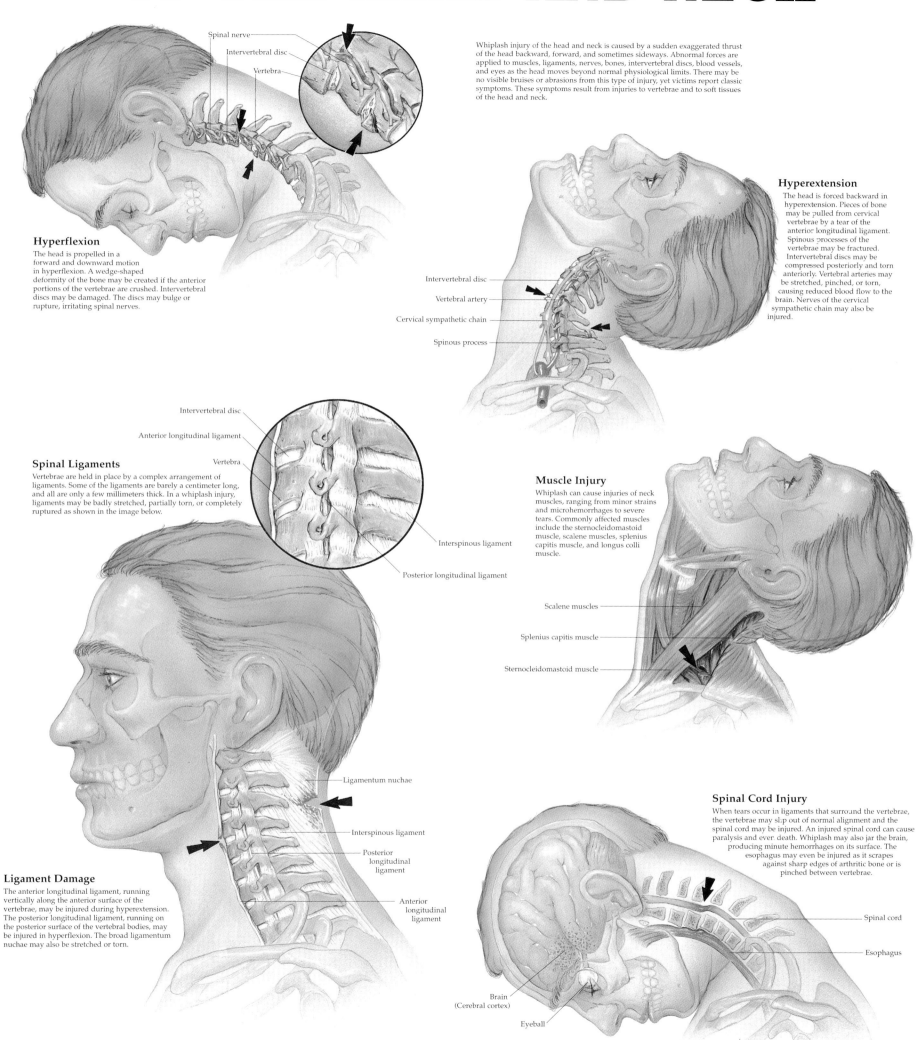

Whiplash injury of the head and neck is caused by a sudden exaggerated thrust of the head backward, forward, and sometimes sideways. Abnormal forces are applied to muscles, ligaments, nerves, bones, intervertebral discs, blood vessels, and eyes as the head moves beyond normal physiological limits. There may be no visible bruises or abrasions from this type of injury, yet victims report classic symptoms. These symptoms result from injuries to vertebrae and to soft tissues of the head and neck.

Spinal nerve
Intervertebral disc
Vertebra

Hyperflexion

The head is propelled in a forward and downward motion in hyperflexion. A wedge-shaped deformity of the bone may be created if the anterior portions of the vertebrae are crushed. Intervertebral discs may be damaged. The discs may bulge or rupture, irritating spinal nerves.

Hyperextension

The head is forced backward in hyperextension. Pieces of bone may be pulled from cervical vertebrae by a tear of the anterior longitudinal ligament. Spinous processes of the vertebrae may be fractured. Intervertebral discs may be compressed posteriorly and torn anteriorly. Vertebral arteries may be stretched, pinched, or torn, causing reduced blood flow to the brain. Nerves of the cervical sympathetic chain may also be injured.

Intervertebral disc
Vertebral artery
Cervical sympathetic chain
Spinous process

Spinal Ligaments

Vertebrae are held in place by a complex arrangement of ligaments. Some of the ligaments are barely a centimeter long, and all are only a few millimeters thick. In a whiplash injury, ligaments may be badly stretched, partially torn, or completely ruptured as shown in the image below.

Intervertebral disc
Anterior longitudinal ligament
Vertebra
Interspinous ligament
Posterior longitudinal ligament

Muscle Injury

Whiplash can cause injuries of neck muscles, ranging from minor strains and microhemorrhages to severe tears. Commonly affected muscles include the sternocleidomastoid muscle, scalene muscles, splenius capitis muscle, and longus colli muscle.

Scalene muscles
Splenius capitis muscle
Sternocleidomastoid muscle

Ligament Damage

The anterior longitudinal ligament, running vertically along the anterior surface of the vertebrae, may be injured during hyperextension. The posterior longitudinal ligament, running on the posterior surface of the vertebral bodies, may be injured in hyperflexion. The broad ligamentum nuchae may also be stretched or torn.

Ligamentum nuchae
Interspinous ligament
Posterior longitudinal ligament
Anterior longitudinal ligament

Spinal Cord Injury

When tears occur in ligaments that surround the vertebrae, the vertebrae may slip out of normal alignment and the spinal cord may be injured. An injured spinal cord can cause paralysis and even death. Whiplash may also jar the brain, producing minute hemorrhages on its surface. The esophagus may even be injured as it scrapes against sharp edges of arthritic bone or is pinched between vertebrae.

Spinal cord
Esophagus
Brain (Cerebral cortex)
Eyeball

9989

Long lasting acid suppression

Mean number of hours in each 24 hours that intragastric pH was above 4 after 1 day and after 5 days of dosing with either PREVACID 30 mg QD, PREVACID 15 mg QD, or omeprazole 20 mg QD in a pharmacodynamic study of 14 healthy subjects[1,7,8]

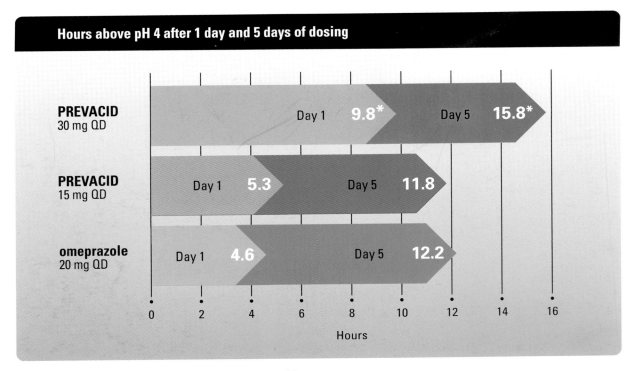

Hours above pH 4 after 1 day and 5 days of dosing

PREVACID 30 mg QD — Day 1 9.8* — Day 5 15.8*
PREVACID 15 mg QD — Day 1 5.3 — Day 5 11.8
omeprazole 20 mg QD — Day 1 4.6 — Day 5 12.2

Hours: 0 2 4 6 8 10 12 14 16

*p<0.001 vs PREVACID 15 mg QD and omeprazole 20 mg QD.

The clinical relevance of these data is unknown.

Prevacid's indications include short-term treatment for healing and symptomatic relief of all grades of erosive esophagitis.

Adverse events reported most frequently with PREVACID were diarrhea, abdominal pain and nausea.

Symptomatic response to therapy does not preclude the presence of gastric malignancy. PREVACID is contraindicated in patients with known hypersensitivity to any component of the formulation. For further information, please see the accompanying complete prescribing information for PREVACID.

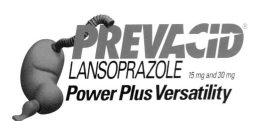

PREVACID®
LANSOPRAZOLE 15 mg and 30 mg
Power Plus Versatility